The Ultimate No Point Weight Loss Cookbook 2025

Low-Carb Delicious, Tasty & Healthy Recipes to Shed Calories while Remaining Zero Count Including a 30-Day Meal Plan

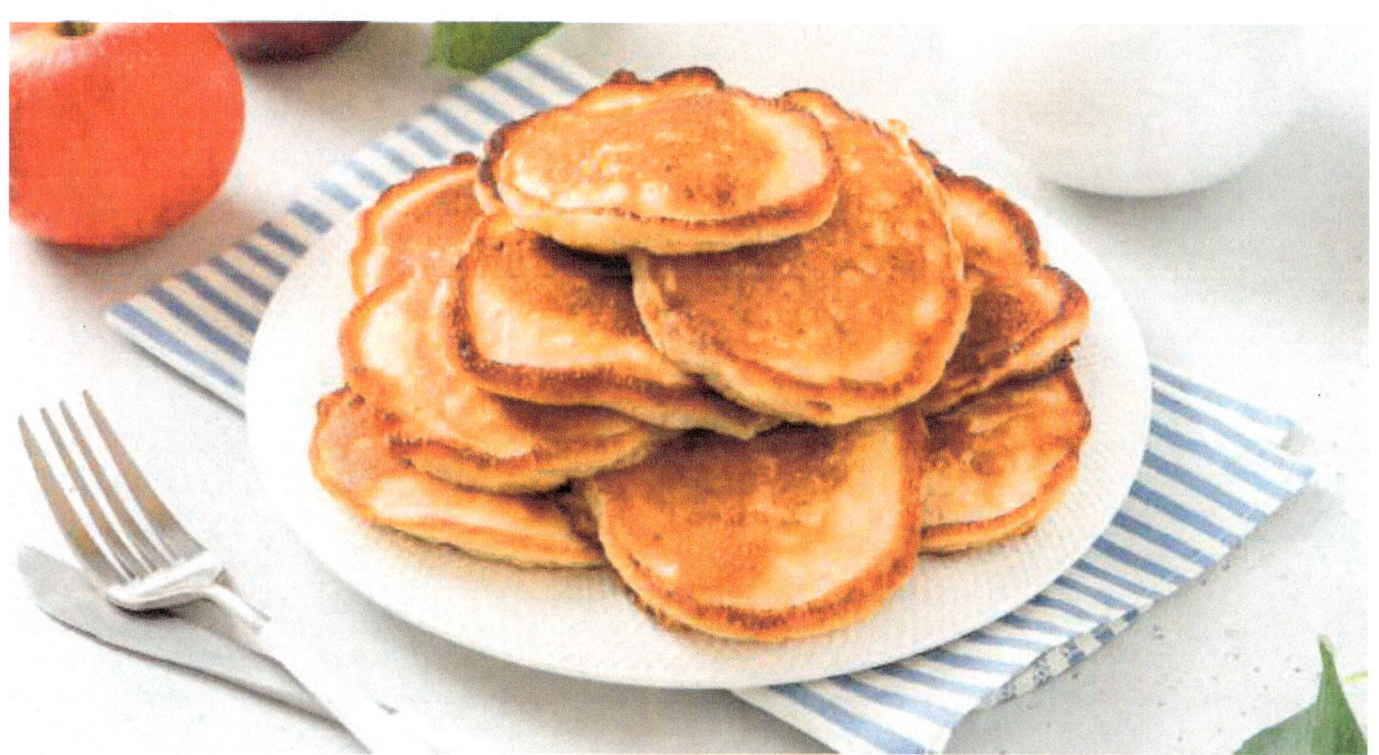

Walter Rivers

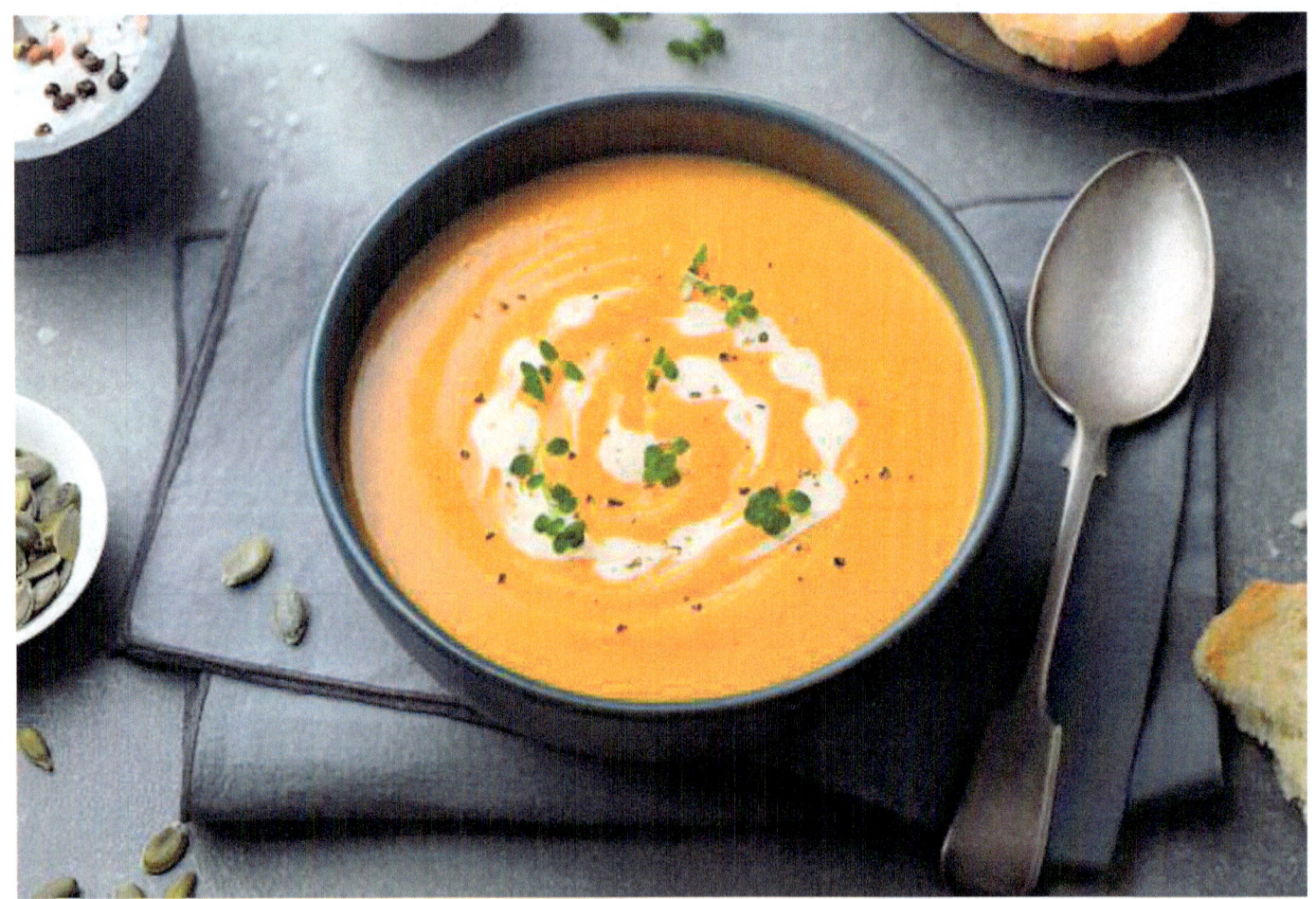

CONTENTS

INTRODUCTION

Welcome to the Zero Point Journey! This cookbook is your guide to exploring zero point foods, where tasty meals and mindful eating go hand in hand. If you've ever thought that healthy eating means giving up your favorite dishes or feeling unsatisfied, think again. This journey is all about savoring food without guilt, and it's a path that leads to both health and happiness.

A while back, I made a friend named Mia. Like many others, she found it hard to enjoy food while staying healthy. One day, she asked me to come over for dinner, excited to share her new recipe—zero point vegetable chili. I was amazed as I took my first bite. It was delicious, filling, and flavorful, but Mia assured me it was guilt-free. She discovered how to turn every meal into a delightful experience, free from concerns about the scale. That night, she told me her secret: using zero point ingredients that let her cook creatively and enjoy her cravings without feeling limited.

This book draws inspiration from people like Mia, who have found that eating well can be straightforward, tasty, and liberating. Here, you'll discover recipes that embrace the same idea—meals you'll eagerly anticipate each day while helping you achieve your weight-loss goals. Prepare to discover new flavors, pick up helpful cooking tips, and whip up meals that make you feel great inside and out. Let's start this journey together!

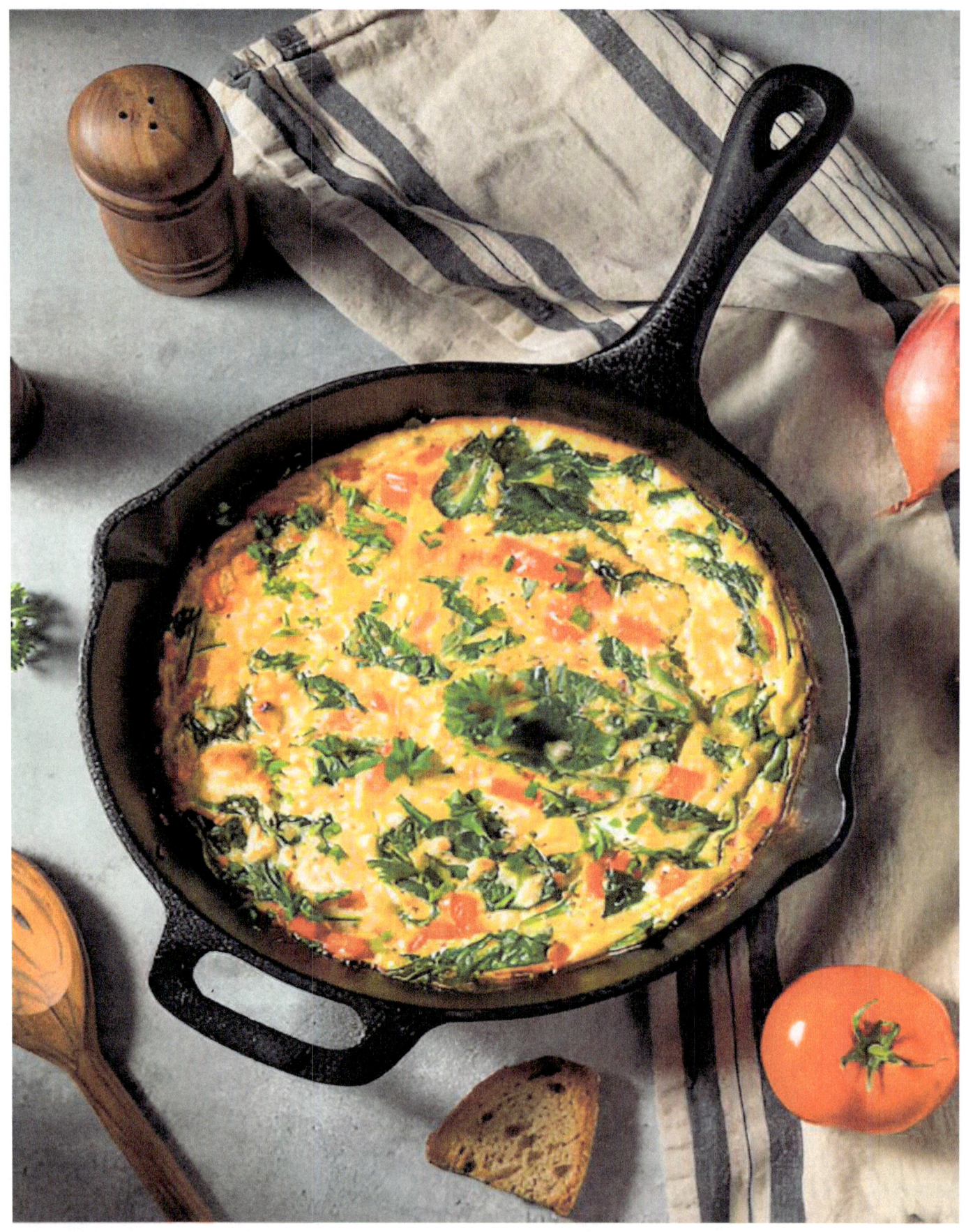

Understanding Zero Point Foods: The Key to Satisfying Weight Loss

Zero point foods are the key to losing weight sustainably while still enjoying your meals. What makes these foods so special? Let's explore this idea and how it can significantly impact your weight-loss journey.

Zero point foods are packed with nutrients, low in calories, and rich in protein, fiber, or water, which makes them very satisfying. You can enjoy a mix of fruits, vegetables, lean proteins, and some whole grains without counting or tracking every bite. By choosing these foods, you can create balanced, enjoyable meals that support your weight-loss goals— without having to do constant calculations.

Zero point foods are great because they help you feel full longer. This can reduce cravings and stop you from snacking on unhealthy choices. A bowl of berries is a refreshing breakfast, and a plate of grilled chicken with roasted vegetables is a hearty, filling dinner. These foods help you feel a sense of plenty instead of limitation, changing your thinking from "I can't have that" to "Look at what I can enjoy!"

This idea is based on the belief that people who can enjoy healthy, unprocessed foods are more likely to stick to their health goals. When you make zero point foods the core of your diet, you create a solid foundation of nutritious meals that energize your body and help you to a healthier lifestyle.

This cookbook features a range of recipes that creatively use zero point foods. Whether you're an experienced chef or a beginner in the kitchen, these meals will support your weight-loss goals while allowing you to enjoy every bite. Enjoy your cooking!

Tips for Staying on Track with Zero Point Recipes

Keeping up with your zero point recipes can be enjoyable and fulfilling when you use the right strategies. Here are some practical tips to help you stay on track, enjoy your meals, and avoid feeling restricted.

Meal Plan for Success

Planning your meals in advance is a great way to help you stay on track. Take some time each week to plan your breakfast, lunch, dinner, and snacks. This approach allows you to select the right ingredients and steer clear of last-minute choices that might result in unhealthy options. Try to regularly cook recipes that freeze nicely, ensuring you always have zero point meals ready to go.

Get Creative with Flavors

Zero point foods are far from boring! Try using herbs, spices, and low-calorie condiments to bring exciting flavors to your meals. Experiment with various cooking methods such as roasting, grilling, or steaming to enhance the natural flavors of your ingredients. A quick squeeze of lemon or a sprinkle of smoked paprika can turn a plain vegetable dish into something vibrant and new.

Incorporate Variety

While zero point foods are plentiful, it's essential to vary your choices to avoid getting tired of the same meals. Incorporate different fruits, vegetables, and lean proteins to make your meals more exciting. For instance, if you typically eat chicken breast, try replacing it with turkey or fish. Using seasonal produce can bring new flavors and make your meals more interesting.

Keep Zero Point Snacks Handy

Not having healthy snacks available is one of the simplest ways to disrupt your eating plan. Fill your fridge and pantry with easy, zero point choices like sliced veggies, hard-boiled eggs, or fresh fruits. These snacks can help satisfy your hunger and prevent you from grabbing high-calorie options when you're in a hurry.

Stay Mindful of Portions

Even though zero point foods can be enjoyed without restriction, paying attention to your body's signals for hunger and fullness is essential. Eating too much, even if it's healthy food, can make you feel tired or uncomfortable. Be mindful of how much you eat. Take your time and really enjoy each bite to ensure you appreciate your meal without going overboard.

Pair Zero point Foods with Healthy Fats and Carbs

Combine zero point foods with healthy fats and complex carbohydrates for balanced and satisfying meals. For example, you can add a bit of avocado to your vegetable salad or enjoy grilled chicken with quinoa. This helps your body get a balanced mix of macronutrients, keeping you full for longer and giving you more energy.

Stay Hydrated

Sometimes, what we think is hunger is really just our body needing water. Drinking water regularly during the day can help reduce unnecessary snacking and keep you feeling full between meals. Enjoy infused waters with simple ingredients like lemon, cucumber, or mint to make hydration fun.

Track Your Progress and Adjust

If you feel like you're losing focus, don't worry! Take a moment to look at your eating habits and make changes if necessary. Writing down what you eat or using an app to track your meals can help you be aware of your food choices and ensure you include enough zero point foods in your diet. Celebrate small victories, such as following your weekly meal plan or experimenting with a new zero point recipe.

Make It a Lifestyle, Not a Diet

Finally, keep in mind that the aim is to achieve weight loss that lasts over time. Zero point foods are more than a quick solution; they're vital parts of a healthy lifestyle you can enjoy for many years. Concentrate on having fun along the way and appreciating the good changes you're making. Embracing the variety and abundance of zero point recipes makes it easier to stay on track.

By using these tips, you'll find it simpler to stick with zero point recipes, stay focused on your weight-loss goals, and enjoy the journey at every stage!

Essential Ingredients and Pantry Staples

Filling your kitchen with the right ingredients is the first step to making tasty zero point meals easily. A well-stocked pantry means you can easily prepare healthy meals, even when short on time. Check out this list of essential ingredients and pantry staples to help you stay on track with your weight-loss journey and make meal prep easy.

Fresh Vegetables: The Foundation of Zero Point Recipes

Vegetables shine in zero point meals, bringing volume, fiber, and flavor. Have a mix of fresh vegetables in your fridge, such as:

- Leafy greens like spinach, kale, and arugula
- Cruciferous veggies like broccoli, cauliflower, and cabbage
- Bell peppers, zucchini, and cucumbers for easy salads and stir-fries
- Carrots, celery, and radishes for snacking or soups
- Tomatoes for salads, sauces, and roasting

These versatile veggies can be used in everything from soups and salads to hearty main dishes.

Fresh and Frozen Fruits: Nature's Sweetness

Fruits are perfect for satisfying your sweet tooth while staying zero points. Keep a mix of fresh and frozen options to add to smoothies, yogurt bowls, or enjoy as a snack:

- Fresh fruits like apples, berries, oranges, and bananas
- Frozen fruits such as mango, pineapple, and mixed berries for smoothies
- Citrus fruits like lemons and limes add a burst of flavor to dishes

Frozen fruits are just as nutritious as fresh and often more convenient when you need a quick, easy option.

Lean Proteins: Building Blocks of a Balanced Diet

Lean proteins are essential for building muscle and keeping you full. Stock up on these zero point protein sources:

- Chicken breasts and turkey (skinless)
- Eggs and egg whites
- Fish like salmon, tilapia, and cod
- Canned tuna or salmon in water
- Tofu and tempeh for plant-based protein options

These proteins can be the base for many meals, from stir-fries to hearty salads.

Canned Goods: Quick and Convenient Additions

Canned goods can be lifesavers when you don't have time for fresh ingredients. Look for low-sodium options when possible:

- Canned beans like black beans, chickpeas, and kidney beans
- Canned tomatoes (diced, crushed, or whole) for soups and sauces
- Canned pumpkin for adding creaminess to soups or making zero point desserts
- Canned vegetables like green beans or corn for quick side dishes

Having these on hand ensures you always have ingredients for a hearty chili or a quick vegetable soup.

Spices, Herbs, and Seasonings: Flavor Without Calories

Spices and herbs are essential for making zero point meals flavorful without increasing calories:

- Dried herbs like oregano, thyme, and basil
- Ground spices like cumin, paprika, chili powder, and turmeric
- Garlic powder, onion powder, and black pepper
- Fresh herbs like cilantro, parsley, and dill
- Low-sodium soy sauce, vinegar (apple cider, balsamic), and hot sauce for an extra kick

These seasonings can transform simple ingredients into vibrant, flavorful dishes that keep you satisfied.

Healthy Cooking Oils and Sprays

Oils may not be zero points, but using them wisely with zero point ingredients can simplify cooking:

- Olive oil spray for roasting veggies or greasing pans
- Zero-calorie non-stick sprays for sautéing
- Fat-free broth (vegetable or chicken) to use in place of oil for cooking or adding flavor to soups

These can be used to keep dishes light while still adding a touch of richness.

Whole Grains: Balanced Carbs for Satisfying Meals

While some grains may not be zero points, adding small amounts can enhance your zero point meals:

- Brown rice, quinoa, or bulgur for hearty salads or sides
- Rolled oats for breakfast or to add to smoothies
- Whole-wheat pasta for pairing with vegetable-based sauces

Adding these in moderate portions alongside zero point foods creates balanced, satisfying meals that keep you full.

Low-Fat Dairy Alternatives

Dairy alternatives can add creaminess without piling on the points:

- Plain Greek yogurt (non-fat) for dips, smoothies, and baking

- Unsweetened almond milk or cashew milk for coffee, cereals, and cooking

- Cottage cheese (low-fat) for adding protein to salads or as a snack

These ingredients can be used to create creamy dressings, add richness to soups, or provide a quick, high-protein snack.

Frozen Vegetables and Proteins: A Backup Plan

Having a variety of frozen vegetables and lean proteins means you can always prepare a zero point meal:

- Frozen spinach, broccoli, and mixed vegetables

- Frozen shrimp or other lean seafood

- Frozen berries and bananas for quick smoothie options

Frozen options are just as nutritious as fresh ones, so always have a meal component ready.

Having these essentials ready means you can whip up delicious, zero point meals anytime, even when life gets hectic. These ingredients allow you to enjoy the simplicity of zero point cooking and concentrate on what truly counts—feeling great and achieving your goals! Enjoy your cooking!

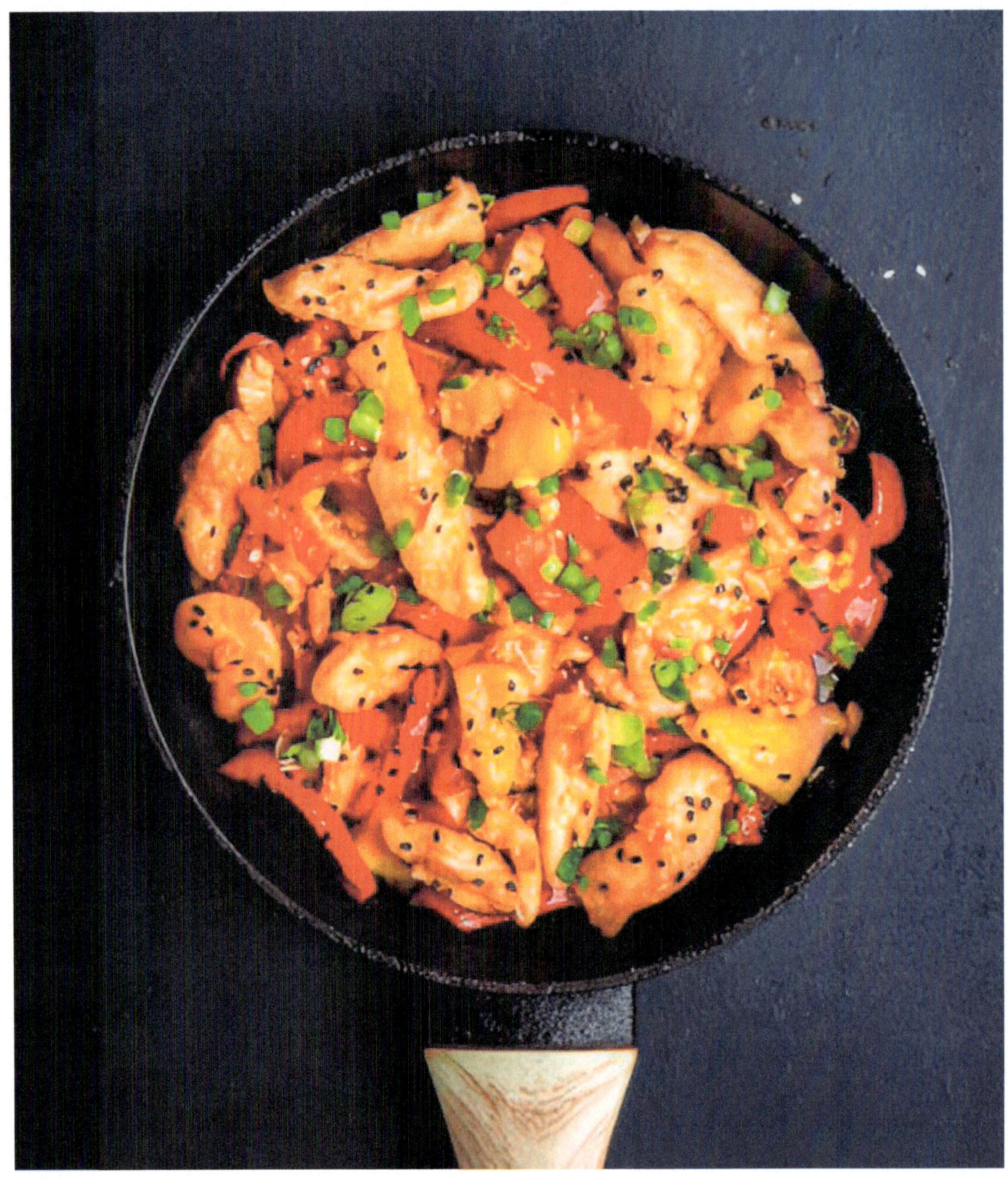

CHAPTER 1: BREAKFAST

Berry Bliss Yogurt Bowl

Time to Prepare: 5 minutes
Cook Time: 0 minutes
Number of Servings: 1

List of Ingredients:

- 1 cup of non-fat plain Greek yogurt
- 1/2 cup of strawberries, sliced
- 1/2 cup of blueberries
- 1/4 cup of raspberries
- 1/2 teaspoon of vanilla extract
- 1/2 teaspoon of cinnamon (optional)

Instructions:

1. In a bowl, mix the non-fat plain Greek yogurt and vanilla extract.
2. Mix well until smooth.
3. Top the yogurt with strawberries, blueberries, and raspberries.
4. Sprinkle with cinnamon if desired.
5. Serve immediately and enjoy!

Nutritional Information (per serving):

- **Total calories:** 100
- **Protein:** 17g
- **Fiber content:** 4g
- **Carbs:** 15g
- **Fats:** 0g

Veggie Omelet

Time to Prepare: 5 minutes
Cook Time: 5 minutes
Number of Servings: 1

List of Ingredients:

- 3 large egg whites
- 1/4 cup of bell peppers, diced (red, yellow, or green)
- 1/4 cup of onion, diced
- 1/4 cup of fresh spinach, chopped
- Salt and pepper, to taste
- Cooking spray

Instructions:

1. Heat a non-stick skillet over medium heat and lightly coat with cooking spray.
2. Add the diced bell peppers and onion. Sauté for 2-3 minutes, until they begin to soften.
3. Add the chopped spinach and cook for an additional 1 minute until wilted.
4. Pour in the egg whites, tilting the skillet to evenly distribute them over the vegetables.
5. Season with salt and pepper to taste.
6. Cook for 2-3 minutes until the egg whites are fully set.
7. Fold the omelet in half and slide it onto a plate.
8. Serve hot.

Nutritional Information (per serving):

- **Total calories:** 60
- **Protein:** 12g
- **Fiber content:** 2g
- **Carbs:** 4g
- **Fats:** 0g

Apple Pie Oatmeal

Time to Prepare: 5 minutes
Cook Time: 5 minutes
Number of Servings: 1

List of Ingredients:

- 1/2 cup of rolled oats
- 1 small apple, diced
- 1/2 teaspoon of ground cinnamon
- 1 cup of water
- 1/2 teaspoon of vanilla extract
- Cooking spray

Instructions:

1. Lightly coat a small saucepan with cooking spray and heat over medium heat.
2. Add the diced apple and cook for 2-3 minutes until slightly softened.
3. Stir in the rolled oats, water, cinnamon, and vanilla extract.
4. Bring the mixture to a boil, then reduce heat and simmer for 3-5 minutes, stirring occasionally, until the oats are cooked and creamy.
5. Serve hot and enjoy.

Nutritional Information (per serving):

- **Total calories:** 150
- **Protein:** 5g
- **Fiber content:** 5g
- **Carbs:** 31g
- **Fats:** 2g

Banana Pancakes

Time to Prepare: 5 minutes
Cook Time: 5 minutes
Number of Servings: 1

List of Ingredients:

- 1 ripe banana
- 2 large eggs
- 1/2 teaspoon of cinnamon (optional)
- Cooking spray

Instructions:

1. In a bowl, mash the ripe banana until smooth.
2. Add the eggs and cinnamon (if using), and whisk until well mixed.
3. Heat a non-stick skillet over medium heat and lightly coat with cooking spray.
4. Pour small portions of the batter onto the skillet to form pancakes.
5. Cook each pancake for 1-2 minutes per side, or until golden brown.
6. Serve hot.

Nutritional Information (per serving):

- **Total calories:** 210
- **Protein:** 12g
- **Fiber content:** 3g
- **Carbs:** 28g
- **Fats:** 5g

Cottage Cheese & Berry Parfait

Time to Prepare: 5 minutes
Cook Time: 0 minutes
Number of Servings: 1

List of Ingredients:

- 1 cup of low-fat cottage cheese
- 1/2 cup of strawberries, sliced
- 1/2 cup of blueberries
- 1/4 teaspoon of cinnamon (optional)

Instructions:

1. In a serving glass or bowl, layer half of the cottage cheese, followed by half of the strawberries and blueberries.
2. Repeat the layers with the remaining cottage cheese and berries.
3. Sprinkle with cinnamon if desired.
4. Serve immediately and enjoy.

Nutritional Information (per serving):

- **Total calories:** 150
- **Protein:** 18g
- **Fiber content:** 3g
- **Carbs:** 12g
- **Fats:** 2g

Green Power Smoothie

Time to Prepare: 5 minutes
Cook Time: 0 minutes
Number of Servings: 1

List of Ingredients:

- 1 cup of fresh spinach
- 1 small banana
- 1/2 green apple, chopped
- 1/2 cup of unsweetened almond milk
- 1/2 cup of water
- Ice cubes (optional)

Instructions:

1. Combine the spinach, banana, green apple, unsweetened almond milk, and water in a blender.
2. Blend until smooth, adding ice cubes if desired for a colder smoothie.
3. Pour into a glass and serve immediately.

Nutritional Information (per serving):

- **Total calories:** 90
- **Protein:** 2g
- **Fiber content:** 4g
- **Carbs:** 21g
- **Fats:** 1g

Spinach and Tomato Egg Muffins

Time to Prepare: 10 minutes
Cook Time: 20 minutes
Number of Servings: 6 (2 muffins per serving)

List of Ingredients:

- 6 large eggs
- 1 cup of fresh spinach, chopped
- 1/2 cup of cherry tomatoes, halved
- Salt and pepper, to taste
- Cooking spray

Instructions:

1. Preheat the oven to 350°F (175°C). Lightly coat a muffin tin with cooking spray.

2. In a mixing bowl, whisk the eggs with salt and pepper.

3. Evenly distribute the chopped spinach and cherry tomato halves into the muffin tin cups of.

4. Pour the egg mixture over the spinach and tomatoes, filling each cup of about 3/4 full.

5. Bake for 18-20 minutes, or until the egg muffins are set and lightly golden on top.

6. Let cool slightly before removing from the tin. Serve warm.

Nutritional Information (per serving):

- **Total calories:** 70
- **Protein:** 10g
- **Fiber content:** 1g
- **Carbs:** 2g
- **Fats:** 3g

Apple Cinnamon Breakfast Bake

Time to Prepare: 10 minutes
Cook Time: 30 minutes
Number of Servings: 4

List of Ingredients:

- 2 cups of rolled oats
- 2 medium apples, diced
- 1 teaspoon of cinnamon
- 1/2 cup of unsweetened applesauce
- 2 cups of unsweetened almond milk
- 1/4 teaspoon of salt
- 1 teaspoon of baking powder
- 1/4 cup of raisins (optional)

Instructions:

1. Preheat the oven to 350°F (175°C) and lightly coat an 8x8 inch baking dish with cooking spray.

2. In a large bowl, mix rolled oats, diced apples, cinnamon, salt, and baking powder.

3. Stir in the unsweetened applesauce and almond milk until well mixed.

4. If using, fold in the raisins.

5. Pour the mixture into the prepared baking dish and spread evenly.

6. Bake for 25-30 minutes, or until the top is golden and set.

7. Allow to cool slightly before cutting into squares. Serve warm.

Nutritional Information (per serving):

- **Total calories:** 150
- **Protein:** 4g
- **Fiber content:** 4g
- **Carbs:** 29g
- **Fats:** 2g

Mushroom and Asparagus Scramble

Time to Prepare: 5 minutes
Cook Time: 10 minutes
Number of Servings: 1

List of Ingredients:

- 3 large egg whites
- 1/2 cup of mushrooms, sliced
- 1/2 cup of asparagus, chopped
- 1/4 cup of onion, diced
- Salt and pepper, to taste
- Cooking spray

Instructions:

1. Heat a non-stick skillet over medium heat and lightly coat with cooking spray.
2. Add the diced onion and sauté for 2-3 minutes until softened.
3. Add the sliced mushrooms and chopped asparagus to the skillet, cooking for an additional 3-4 minutes until the vegetables are tender.
4. Pour in the egg whites and season with salt and pepper.
5. Cook, stirring gently, until the egg whites are fully set.
6. Serve immediately.

Nutritional Information (per serving):

- **Total calories:** 60
- **Protein:** 11g
- **Fiber content:** 2g
- **Carbs:** 4g
- **Fats:** 0g

Mixed Berry Chia Pudding

Time to Prepare: 5 minutes
Cook Time: 0 minutes
Number of Servings: 2

List of Ingredients:

- 1/4 cup of chia seeds
- 1 cup of unsweetened almond milk
- 1/2 cup of mixed berries (strawberries, blueberries, raspberries)
- 1 teaspoon of vanilla extract (optional)
- Sweetener of choice (optional, adjust to taste)

Instructions:

1. In a medium bowl, mix chia seeds, unsweetened almond milk, vanilla extract, and sweetener (if using).
2. Stir well to mix, ensuring there are no clumps of chia seeds.
3. Let the mixture sit for about 5 minutes, then stir again to prevent clumping.
4. Cover and refrigerate for at least 2 hours, or overnight, to allow the pudding to thicken.
5. Once set, stir again and divide the chia pudding into serving bowls.
6. Top with mixed berries before serving.

Nutritional Information (per serving):

- **Total calories:** 120
- **Protein:** 4g
- **Fiber content:** 8g
- **Carbs:** 16g
- **Fats:** 6g

Tropical Fruit Salad

Time to Prepare: 10 minutes
Cook Time: 0 minutes
Number of Servings: 4

List of Ingredients:

- 1 cup of fresh pineapple, diced
- 1 cup of fresh mango, diced
- 1 cup of fresh papaya, diced
- 1/2 cup of strawberries, sliced (optional)
- Juice of 1 lime
- Fresh mint leaves for garnish (optional)

Instructions:

1. In a large bowl, mix the diced pineapple, mango, papaya, and sliced strawberries (if using).
2. Drizzle the lime juice over the fruit and gently toss to mix.
3. Let the salad sit for a few minutes to allow the flavors to meld.
4. Serve in individual bowls and garnish with fresh mint leaves if desired.

Nutritional Information (per serving):

- **Total calories:** 60
- **Protein:** 1g
- **Fiber content:** 3g
- **Carbs:** 15g
- **Fats:** 0g

Spiced Pumpkin Puree with Yogurt

Time to Prepare: 5 minutes
Cook Time: 0 minutes
Number of Servings: 2

List of Ingredients:

- 1 cup of canned pure pumpkin (not pumpkin pie filling)
- 1/2 cup of non-fat plain Greek yogurt
- 1 teaspoon of pumpkin pie spice (or a mix of cinnamon, nutmeg, and ginger)
- 1 teaspoon of maple syrup or sweetener of choice (optional)
- 1/4 teaspoon of vanilla extract (optional)

Instructions:

1. In a medium bowl, mix the canned pumpkin, Greek yogurt, pumpkin pie spice, maple syrup (if using), and vanilla extract (if using).
2. Mix well until smooth and evenly mixed.
3. Serve immediately or refrigerate for up to 1 hour to chill.
4. Divide into bowls and enjoy.

Nutritional Information (per serving):

- **Total calories:** 90
- **Protein:** 8g
- **Fiber content:** 3g
- **Carbs:** 12g
- **Fats:** 0g

Roasted Red Pepper and Spinach Egg White Cups

Time to Prepare: 10 minutes
Cook Time: 20 minutes
Number of Servings: 6

List of Ingredients:

- 6 large egg whites
- 1/2 cup of roasted red peppers, diced
- 1 cup of fresh spinach, chopped
- 1/4 cup of onion, diced
- Salt and pepper, to taste
- Cooking spray

Instructions:

1. Preheat the oven to 350°F (175°C) and lightly coat a muffin tin with cooking spray.
2. In a mixing bowl, whisk the egg whites with salt and pepper.
3. In a skillet over medium heat, sauté the diced onion until softened, about 3-4 minutes.
4. Add the chopped spinach and diced roasted red peppers to the skillet, cooking for an additional 2-3 minutes until the spinach is wilted.
5. Evenly distribute the vegetable mixture into the muffin tin cups of.
6. Pour the egg white mixture over the vegetables, filling each cup of about 3/4 full.
7. Bake for 15-20 minutes, or until the egg whites are set and slightly golden.
8. Allow to cool slightly before removing from the tin. Serve warm.

Nutritional Information (per serving):

- **Total calories:** 40
- **Protein:** 8g
- **Fiber content:** 1g
- **Carbs:** 2g
- **Fats:** 0g

Banana-Berry Smoothie Bowl

Time to Prepare: 5 minutes
Cook Time: 0 minutes
Number of Servings: 1

List of Ingredients:

- 1 ripe banana, frozen
- 1/2 cup of mixed berries (strawberries, blueberries, raspberries)
- 1/2 cup of unsweetened almond milk
- 1/2 teaspoon of vanilla extract (optional)
- Toppings (e.g., additional berries, sliced banana, or chia seeds – optional, not included in nutritional info)

Instructions:

1. In a blender, mix the frozen banana, mixed berries, unsweetened almond milk, and vanilla extract (if using).
2. Blend until smooth and creamy.
3. Pour the smoothie into a bowl and add your choice of toppings if desired.
4. Serve immediately.

Nutritional Information (per serving):

- **Total calories:** 150
- **Protein:** 2g
- **Fiber content:** 5g
- **Carbs:** 35g
- **Fats:** 1g

Egg White and Salsa Wrap

Time to Prepare: 5 minutes
Cook Time: 5 minutes
Number of Servings: 1

List of Ingredients:

- 3 large egg whites
- 1/4 cup of salsa (fresh or store-bought)
- 2 large lettuce leaves (for wrapping)
- Salt and pepper, to taste
- Cooking spray

Instructions:

1. Heat a non-stick skillet over medium heat and lightly coat with cooking spray.
2. In a bowl, whisk the egg whites with salt and pepper.
3. Pour the egg whites into the skillet and cook for 2-3 minutes, stirring gently until fully set.
4. Remove from heat and stir in the salsa.
5. Place the egg white and salsa mixture onto the center of each lettuce leaf.
6. Fold the sides of the lettuce leaves over the filling and serve as a wrap.

Nutritional Information (per serving):

- **Total calories:** 60
- **Protein:** 11g
- **Fiber content:** 1g
- **Carbs:** 3g
- **Fats:** 0g

Pear and Ginger Smoothie

Time to Prepare: 5 minutes
Cook Time: 0 minutes
Number of Servings: 1

List of Ingredients:

- 1 ripe pear, cored and chopped
- 1/2 inch piece of fresh ginger, peeled and grated
- 1/2 cup of unsweetened almond milk
- 1/4 cup of water
- Ice cubes (optional)

Instructions:

1. In a blender, mix the chopped pear, grated ginger, unsweetened almond milk, and water.
2. Blend until smooth, adding ice cubes if desired for a colder smoothie.
3. Pour into a glass and serve immediately.

Nutritional Information (per serving):

- **Total calories:** 100
- **Protein:** 1g
- **Fiber content:** 5g
- **Carbs:** 24g
- **Fats:** 1g

Baked Apple Slices with Cinnamon

Time to Prepare: 10 minutes
Cook Time: 20 minutes
Number of Servings: 4

List of Ingredients:

- 4 medium apples, cored and sliced
- 1 teaspoon of cinnamon
- 1 tablespoon lemon juice
- Cooking spray or parchment paper

Instructions:

1. Preheat the oven to 350°F (175°C) and line a baking sheet with parchment paper or lightly coat with cooking spray.
2. In a large bowl, toss the apple slices with lemon juice and cinnamon until evenly coated.
3. Arrange the apple slices in a single layer on the prepared baking sheet.
4. Bake for 15-20 minutes, or until the apples are tender and slightly caramelized.
5. Remove from the oven and let cool slightly before serving.

Nutritional Information (per serving):

- **Total calories:** 80
- **Protein:** 0g
- **Fiber content:** 3g
- **Carbs:** 22g
- **Fats:** 0g

Lemon and Blueberry Overnight Oats

Time to Prepare: 10 minutes
Cook Time: 0 minutes
Number of Servings: 1

List of Ingredients:

- 1/2 cup of plain rolled oats
- 1/2 cup of unsweetened almond milk
- 1/2 cup of fresh blueberries
- Zest of 1 lemon
- 1 tablespoon lemon juice
- 1 teaspoon of sweetener of choice (optional)

Instructions:

1. In a jar or a bowl, mix the rolled oats, almond milk, lemon zest, lemon juice, and sweetener (if using).
2. Stir well to mix, ensuring the oats are fully submerged in the liquid.
3. Gently fold in the fresh blueberries.
4. Cover and refrigerate overnight (or at least 4 hours) to allow the oats to absorb the liquid.
5. Stir before serving and enjoy cold.

Nutritional Information (per serving):

- **Total calories:** 200
- **Protein:** 6g
- **Fiber content:** 8g
- **Carbs:** 36g
- **Fats:** 4g

Grilled Peach and Greek Yogurt Bowl

Time to Prepare: 10 minutes
Cook Time: 5 minutes
Number of Servings: 1

List of Ingredients:

- 1 ripe peach, halved and pitted
- 1/2 cup of non-fat plain Greek yogurt
- 1 teaspoon of honey or sweetener of choice (optional)
- 1/4 teaspoon of cinnamon (optional)
- Fresh mint leaves for garnish (optional)

Instructions:

1. Preheat a grill or grill pan over medium heat.
2. Lightly coat the cut side of the peach halves with cooking spray.
3. Place the peaches cut-side down on the grill and cook for about 3-5 minutes, until grill marks appear and the peaches are tender.
4. Remove the peaches from the grill and let cool slightly.
5. In a bowl, spoon the Greek yogurt and drizzle with honey or sweetener (if using). Sprinkle with cinnamon, if desired.
6. Top the yogurt with the grilled peach halves and garnish with fresh mint leaves, if desired.
7. Serve immediately.

Nutritional Information (per serving):

- **Total calories:** 150
- **Protein:** 11g
- **Fiber content:** 2g
- **Carbs:** 22g
- **Fats:** 0g

Herb and Tomato Frittata

Time to Prepare: 10 minutes
Cook Time: 15 minutes
Number of Servings: 4

List of Ingredients:

- 6 large egg whites
- 1 cup of cherry tomatoes, halved
- 1/2 cup of fresh spinach, chopped
- 1/4 cup of onion, diced
- 1 teaspoon of dried Italian herbs (or a mix of basil, oregano, and thyme)
- Salt and pepper, to taste
- Cooking spray

Instructions:

1. Preheat the oven to 375°F (190°C) and lightly coat a 9-inch pie dish or oven-safe skillet with cooking spray.
2. In a mixing bowl, whisk the egg whites with salt, pepper, and dried herbs.
3. In a skillet over medium heat, sauté the diced onion until softened, about 3 minutes.
4. Add the cherry tomatoes and chopped spinach to the skillet, cooking for an additional 2-3 minutes until the spinach is wilted.
5. Pour the egg white mixture over the vegetables in the skillet, gently stirring to mix.
6. Cook on the stove for 2-3 minutes until the edges start to set, then transfer the skillet to the preheated oven.
7. Bake for 10-12 minutes, or until the frittata is set in the center and lightly golden.
8. Remove from the oven, let cool slightly, and cut into wedges to serve.

Nutritional Information (per serving):

- **Total calories:** 50
- **Protein:** 10g
- **Fiber content:** 1g
- **Carbs:** 3g
- **Fats:** 0g

CHAPTER 2: LUNCH

Mediterranean Chickpea Salad

Time to Prepare: 15 minutes
Cook Time: 0 minutes
Number of Servings: 4

List of Ingredients:

- 1 can (15 oz) chickpeas, drained and rinsed
- 1 cup of cherry tomatoes, halved
- 1/2 cucumber, diced
- 1/4 red onion, finely chopped
- 1/4 cup of parsley, chopped
- Juice of 1 lemon
- 1 tablespoon red wine vinegar
- Salt and pepper, to taste
- 1/2 teaspoon of dried oregano

Instructions:

1. In a large bowl, mix the chickpeas, cherry tomatoes, cucumber, red onion, and parsley.
2. In a separate small bowl, whisk together the lemon juice, red wine vinegar, salt, pepper, and dried oregano.
3. Pour the dressing over the salad and toss gently to mix.
4. Let the salad sit for 5-10 minutes to allow the flavors to meld before serving.

Nutritional Information (per serving):

- **Total calories:** 120
- **Protein:** 6g
- **Fiber content:** 6g
- **Carbs:** 18g
- **Fats:** 1g

Tuna and Cucumber Lettuce Wraps

Time to Prepare: 10 minutes
Cook Time: 0 minutes
Number of Servings: 2

List of Ingredients:

- 1 can (5 oz) tuna in water, drained
- 1/4 cup of plain non-fat Greek yogurt
- 1 tablespoon Dijon mustard
- 1/4 cup of celery, finely chopped
- 1/4 cup of red onion, finely chopped
- 1 tablespoon lemon juice
- Salt and pepper, to taste
- 4 large lettuce leaves (such as romaine or butter lettuce)
- 1/2 cucumber, sliced (for additional crunch)

Instructions:

1. In a bowl, mix the drained tuna, Greek yogurt, Dijon mustard, chopped celery, red onion, lemon juice, salt, and pepper. Mix until well mixed.
2. Lay the large lettuce leaves flat on a clean surface.
3. Spoon the tuna mixture evenly onto each lettuce leaf.
4. Top with cucumber slices for extra crunch.
5. Roll the lettuce leaves up to form wraps and serve immediately.

Nutritional Information (per serving):

- **Total calories:** 140
- **Protein:** 22g
- **Fiber content:** 2g
- **Carbs:** 4g
- **Fats:** 2g

Spicy Black Bean Soup

Time to Prepare: 10 minutes
Cook Time: 30 minutes
Number of Servings: 4

List of Ingredients:

- 2 cans (15 oz each) black beans, drained and rinsed
- 1 can (14.5 oz) diced tomatoes with green chilies
- 1 small onion, chopped
- 2 cloves garlic, minced
- 1 cup of vegetable broth (low-sodium)
- 1 teaspoon of ground cumin
- 1 teaspoon of chili powder
- 1/2 teaspoon of cayenne pepper (adjust to taste)
- Salt and pepper, to taste
- 1 tablespoon lime juice
- Fresh cilantro for garnish (optional)

Instructions:

1. In a large pot, sauté the chopped onion and minced garlic over medium heat until softened, about 5 minutes.
2. Add the diced tomatoes with green chilies, black beans, vegetable broth, ground cumin, chili powder, cayenne pepper, salt, and pepper.
3. Bring the mixture to a boil, then reduce the heat and let it simmer for 20 minutes, stirring occasionally.
4. Use an immersion blender to partially blend the soup for a creamier texture, or transfer a portion to a blender and blend until smooth. (Be careful with hot liquids!)
5. Stir in lime juice and adjust seasoning if needed.
6. Serve hot, garnished with fresh cilantro if desired.

Nutritional Information (per serving):

- **Total calories:** 150
- **Protein:** 9g
- **Fiber content:** 7g
- **Carbs:** 27g
- **Fats:** 0g

Zucchini Noodles with Tomato and Basil

Time to Prepare: 10 minutes
Cook Time: 10 minutes
Number of Servings: 2

List of Ingredients:

- 2 medium zucchinis, spiralized into noodles
- 2 cups of cherry tomatoes, halved
- 2 cloves garlic, minced
- 1 tablespoon olive oil (optional; can be replaced with cooking spray for zero points)
- 1/4 cup of fresh basil, chopped
- Salt and pepper, to taste
- 1/4 teaspoon of red pepper flakes (optional)

Instructions:

1. In a large skillet, heat olive oil over medium heat (or use cooking spray).
2. Add minced garlic and cherry tomatoes to the skillet. Sauté for 3-4 minutes until the tomatoes start to soften.
3. Add the spiralized zucchini noodles to the skillet and toss to mix with the tomato mixture. Cook for an additional 3-5 minutes until the zucchini is tender but still slightly crunchy.
4. Season with salt, pepper, and red pepper flakes (if using).
5. Remove from heat and stir in the fresh basil.
6. Serve immediately, garnished with additional basil if desired.

Nutritional Information (per serving):

- **Total calories:** 80
- **Protein:** 3g
- **Fiber content:** 3g
- **Carbs:** 15g
- **Fats:** 2g

Rainbow Veggie Wraps

Time to Prepare: 15 minutes
Cook Time: 0 minutes
Number of Servings: 4

List of Ingredients:

- 8 large cabbage leaves
- 1 cup of bell peppers, thinly sliced (mix of red, yellow, and green)
- 1 cup of cucumber, julienned
- 1 cup of carrots, shredded
- 1 cup of purple cabbage, shredded
- 1/2 cup of shredded lettuce
- 1/4 cup of fresh cilantro, chopped
- 1 tablespoon lime juice
- Salt and pepper, to taste
- Optional: 1/4 cup of hummus or yogurt-based dressing for dipping

Instructions:

1. Carefully remove the cabbage leaves from the head and rinse under cold water.
2. Pat the leaves dry and lay them flat on a clean surface.
3. In a large bowl, mix the bell peppers, cucumber, carrots, purple cabbage, shredded lettuce, cilantro, lime juice, salt, and pepper. Toss to mix well.
4. Place a portion of the veggie mixture in the center of each cabbage leaf.
5. Fold in the sides of the leaf and roll it up tightly to form a wrap.
6. Repeat with the remaining leaves and filling.
7. Serve immediately with optional hummus or yogurt-based dressing for dipping.

Nutritional Information (per serving):

- **Total calories:** 50
- **Protein:** 2g
- **Fiber content:** 5g
- **Carbs:** 10g
- **Fats:** 0g

Shrimp and Mango Salad

Time to Prepare: 15 minutes
Cook Time: 5 minutes
Number of Servings: 2

List of Ingredients:

- 8 oz cooked shrimp, peeled and deveined
- 1 ripe mango, diced
- 2 cups of mixed greens (spinach, arugula, etc.)
- 1/2 red bell pepper, diced
- 1/4 red onion, thinly sliced
- 1/4 cup of fresh cilantro, chopped
- Juice of 1 lime
- Salt and pepper, to taste

Instructions:

1. In a large bowl, mix the cooked shrimp, diced mango, mixed greens, red bell pepper, red onion, and cilantro.
2. Drizzle the lime juice over the salad and season with salt and pepper.
3. Toss gently to mix, ensuring the ingredients are well mixed.
4. Serve immediately.

Nutritional Information (per serving):

- **Total calories:** 180
- **Protein:** 22g
- **Fiber content:** 3g
- **Carbs:** 14g
- **Fats:** 3g

Cabbage Soup with Lean Turkey

Time to Prepare: 10 minutes
Cook Time: 30 minutes
Number of Servings: 6

List of Ingredients:

- 1 lb lean ground turkey
- 4 cups of cabbage, chopped
- 1 can (14.5 oz) diced tomatoes (no added sugar)
- 1 cup of carrots, diced
- 1 cup of celery, diced
- 1 small onion, chopped
- 4 cups of low-sodium vegetable broth
- 2 cloves garlic, minced
- 1 teaspoon of dried oregano
- 1 teaspoon of paprika
- Salt and pepper, to taste
- 1 tablespoon fresh parsley, chopped (for garnish)

Instructions:

1. In a large pot, brown the lean ground turkey over medium heat until fully cooked. Drain any excess fat.

2. Add the chopped onion and garlic to the pot, sautéing for 2-3 minutes until the onion is translucent.

3. Stir in the diced tomatoes, cabbage, carrots, celery, vegetable broth, dried oregano, paprika, salt, and pepper.

4. Bring the mixture to a boil, then reduce the heat and let it simmer for about 20 minutes, or until the vegetables are tender.

5. Taste and adjust seasoning if necessary.

6. Serve hot, garnished with fresh parsley.

Nutritional Information (per serving):

- **Total calories:** 150
- **Protein:** 20g
- **Fiber content:** 4g
- **Carbs:** 10g
- **Fats:** 4g

Grilled Veggie Skewers with Lemon

Time to Prepare: 15 minutes
Cook Time: 10 minutes
Number of Servings: 4

List of Ingredients:

- 2 bell peppers (any color), cut into 1-inch pieces
- 1 medium zucchini, sliced into rounds
- 1 medium yellow squash, sliced into rounds
- 1 red onion, cut into wedges
- 1 cup of cherry tomatoes
- 1 tablespoon olive oil (optional; can be replaced with cooking spray for zero)
- Juice of 1 lemon
- 1 teaspoon of garlic powder
- 1 teaspoon of dried oregano
- Salt and pepper, to taste
- Wooden or metal skewers

Instructions:

1. Preheat the grill to medium-high heat.

2. If using wooden skewers, soak them in water for 30 minutes to prevent burning.

3. In a large bowl, mix the bell peppers, zucchini, yellow squash, red onion, and cherry tomatoes.

4. Drizzle with olive oil (if using), lemon juice, garlic powder, oregano, salt, and pepper. Toss to coat the veggies evenly.

5. Thread the vegetables onto the skewers, alternating colors for a vibrant presentation.

6. Place the skewers on the preheated grill and cook for about 10 minutes, turning occasionally, until the veggies are tender and have grill marks.

7. Remove from the grill and serve immediately.

Nutritional Information (per serving):

- **Total calories:** 60
- **Protein:** 2g
- **Fiber content:** 3g
- **Carbs:** 12g
- **Fats:** 2g

Spinach, Apple, and Walnut Salad

Time to Prepare: 10 minutes
Cook Time: 0 minutes
Number of Servings: 4

List of Ingredients:

- 6 cups of fresh spinach, washed and dried
- 1 medium apple, thinly sliced (any variety)
- 1/2 cup of walnuts, chopped
- 1/4 cup of red onion, thinly sliced
- 1/4 cup of balsamic vinegar
- 1 tablespoon Dijon mustard
- Salt and pepper, to taste

Instructions:

1. In a large salad bowl, mix the fresh spinach, sliced apple, chopped walnuts, and red onion.
2. In a small bowl, whisk together the balsamic vinegar, Dijon mustard, salt, and pepper until well mixed.
3. Drizzle the dressing over the salad and toss gently to coat all ingredients.
4. Serve immediately.

Nutritional Information (per serving):

- **Total calories:** 150
- **Protein:** 4g
- **Fiber content:** 4g
- **Carbs:** 18g
- **Fats:** 8g

Cucumber, Tomato, and Red Onion Salad

Time to Prepare: 10 minutes
Cook Time: 0 minutes
Number of Servings: 4

List of Ingredients:

- 2 large cucumbers, diced
- 2 cups of cherry tomatoes, halved
- 1/2 red onion, thinly sliced
- 1/4 cup of fresh parsley, chopped
- 2 tablespoons red wine vinegar
- 1 tablespoon olive oil (optional; can be replaced with cooking spray for zero points)
- Salt and pepper, to taste

Instructions:

1. In a large mixing bowl, mix the diced cucumbers, cherry tomatoes, red onion, and fresh parsley.
2. In a small bowl, whisk together the red wine vinegar, olive oil (if using), salt, and pepper.
3. Drizzle the dressing over the salad and toss gently to mix.
4. Serve immediately or refrigerate for 30 minutes to allow the flavors to meld.

Nutritional Information (per serving):

- **Total calories:** 50
- **Protein:** 2g
- **Fiber content:** 3g
- **Carbs:** 10g
- **Fats:** 2g

Butternut Squash Soup

Time to Prepare: 10 minutes
Cook Time: 30 minutes
Number of Servings: 4

List of Ingredients:

- 1 medium butternut squash, peeled and cubed
- 1 medium onion, chopped
- 2 cloves garlic, minced
- 4 cups of low-sodium vegetable broth
- 1 teaspoon of ground cinnamon
- 1/2 teaspoon of ground nutmeg
- Salt and pepper, to taste
- 1 tablespoon olive oil (optional; can be replaced with cooking spray for zero points)
- Fresh parsley, for garnish (optional)

Instructions:

1. In a large pot, heat the olive oil (if using) over medium heat. Add the chopped onion and garlic, sautéing until the onion is translucent, about 3-4 minutes.
2. Add the cubed butternut squash, vegetable broth, cinnamon, nutmeg, salt, and pepper to the pot.
3. Bring the mixture to a boil, then reduce heat and let it simmer for about 20 minutes, or until the butternut squash is tender.
4. Remove from heat and use an immersion blender to puree the soup until smooth. (Alternatively, transfer to a blender in batches.)
5. Taste and adjust seasoning if necessary. Garnish with fresh parsley if desired and serve hot.

Nutritional Information (per serving):

- **Total calories:** 90
- **Protein:** 2g
- **Fiber content:** 3g
- **Carbs:** 20g
- **Fats:** 2g

Baked Bell Pepper and Tomato Casserole

Time to Prepare: 15 minutes
Cook Time: 35 minutes
Number of Servings: 4

List of Ingredients:

- 4 large bell peppers (any color), halved and seeds removed
- 2 cups of diced tomatoes (fresh or canned, no added sugar)
- 1 medium onion, chopped
- 2 cloves garlic, minced
- 1 cup of cooked quinoa or brown rice
- 1 teaspoon of dried Italian herbs (oregano, basil, thyme)
- Salt and pepper, to taste
- 1/4 cup of fresh parsley, chopped (for garnish)
- Cooking spray

Instructions:

1. Preheat the oven to 375°F (190°C). Lightly spray a baking dish with cooking spray.
2. In a skillet over medium heat, sauté the chopped onion and garlic until softened, about 3-4 minutes.
3. In a large bowl, mix the diced tomatoes, cooked quinoa or brown rice, sautéed onion and garlic, dried herbs, salt, and pepper.
4. Stuff each bell pepper half with the tomato mixture and place them in the prepared baking dish.
5. Cover the dish with aluminum foil and bake for 25 minutes. Remove the foil and bake for an additional 10 minutes, until the peppers are tender.
6. Remove from the oven and garnish with fresh parsley before serving.

Nutritional Information (per serving):

- **Total calories:** 120
- **Protein:** 4g
- **Fiber content:** 5g
- **Carbs:** 25g
- **Fats:** 1g

Roasted Cauliflower and Chickpea Bowl

Time to Prepare: 15 minutes
Cook Time: 25 minutes
Number of Servings: 4

List of Ingredients:

- 1 head of cauliflower, cut into florets
- 1 can (15 oz) chickpeas, drained and rinsed
- 2 tablespoons olive oil (optional; can be replaced with cooking spray for zero)
- 1 teaspoon of paprika
- 1 teaspoon of garlic powder
- 1/2 teaspoon of cumin
- Salt and pepper, to taste
- 4 cups of mixed greens (spinach, arugula, or your choice)
- 1/4 cup of tahini or your favorite dressing (optional)

Instructions:

1. Preheat the oven to 425°F (220°C). Line a baking sheet with parchment paper.
2. In a large bowl, toss the cauliflower florets and chickpeas with olive oil (if using), paprika, garlic powder, cumin, salt, and pepper until well coated.
3. Spread the mixture evenly on the prepared baking sheet. Roast in the oven for 20-25 minutes, or until the cauliflower is golden brown and tender, stirring halfway through.
4. While the cauliflower and chickpeas are roasting, prepare the mixed greens in serving bowls.
5. Once roasted, remove from the oven and let cool slightly before topping the mixed greens with the roasted cauliflower and chickpeas.
6. Drizzle with tahini or your choice of dressing, if desired, and serve warm.

Nutritional Information (per serving):

- **Total calories:** 180
- **Protein:** 6g
- **Fiber content:** 8g
- **Carbs:** 30g
- **Fats:** 6g

Grilled Chicken Breast with Citrus Salad

Time to Prepare: 15 minutes
Cook Time: 20 minutes
Number of Servings: 4

List of Ingredients:

- 4 boneless, skinless chicken breasts
- 2 tablespoons olive oil (optional; can be replaced with cooking spray for zero points)
- 1 teaspoon of garlic powder
- 1 teaspoon of paprika
- Salt and pepper, to taste
- 2 cups of mixed greens (spinach, arugula, or your choice)
- 1 cup of orange segments (fresh or canned in juice)
- 1 cup of grapefruit segments (fresh or canned in juice)
- 1/4 red onion, thinly sliced
- 1/4 cup of balsamic vinegar (for dressing)

Instructions:

1. Preheat the grill to medium-high heat. If using olive oil, brush the chicken breasts with olive oil and season with garlic powder, paprika, salt, and pepper.
2. Grill the chicken breasts for about 6-7 minutes per side, or until cooked through and the internal temperature reaches 165°F (75°C). Remove from the grill and let rest for a few minutes before slicing.
3. In a large bowl, mix the mixed greens, orange segments, grapefruit segments, and red onion.
4. Slice the grilled chicken and arrange it on top of the salad. Drizzle with balsamic vinegar before serving.

Nutritional Information (per serving):

- **Total calories:** 230
- **Protein:** 30g
- **Fiber content:** 3g
- **Carbs:** 10g
- **Fats:** 10g

Carrot and Ginger Soup

Time to Prepare: 10 minutes
Cook Time: 30 minutes
Number of Servings: 4

List of Ingredients:

- 4 large carrots, peeled and chopped
- 1 medium onion, chopped
- 2 cloves garlic, minced
- 1 tablespoon fresh ginger, grated
- 4 cups of low-sodium vegetable broth
- 1 tablespoon olive oil (optional; can be replaced with cooking spray for zero points)
- Salt and pepper, to taste
- 1/4 cup of coconut milk (optional, for creaminess)
- Fresh cilantro, for garnish (optional)

Instructions:

1. In a large pot, heat the olive oil (if using) over medium heat. Add the chopped onion and garlic, sautéing until softened, about 3-4 minutes.

2. Add the chopped carrots and grated ginger to the pot, stirring for another 2 minutes.

3. Pour in the vegetable broth and bring the mixture to a boil. Reduce heat and let it simmer for 20 minutes, or until the carrots are tender.

4. Use an immersion blender to puree the soup until smooth. (Alternatively, carefully transfer to a blender in batches.)

5. If desired, stir in coconut milk for added creaminess. Season with salt and pepper to taste.

6. Serve hot, garnished with fresh cilantro if desired.

Nutritional Information (per serving):

- **Total calories:** 90
- **Protein:** 2g
- **Fiber content:** 4g
- **Carbs:** 19g
- **Fats:** 3g

Sweet and Sour Cabbage Slaw

Time to Prepare: 15 minutes
Cook Time: 0 minutes
Number of Servings: 4

List of Ingredients:

- 4 cups of green cabbage, thinly sliced
- 1 cup of carrots, grated
- 1/2 red bell pepper, thinly sliced
- 1/2 cup of apple cider vinegar
- 2 tablespoons sugar substitute (like Stevia or Splenda)
- 1 tablespoon olive oil (optional; can be replaced with cooking spray for zero points)
- Salt and pepper, to taste
- 1/4 cup of chopped fresh parsley (optional)

Instructions:

1. In a large bowl, mix the sliced cabbage, grated carrots, and sliced red bell pepper.

2. In a separate small bowl, whisk together the apple cider vinegar, sugar substitute, olive oil (if using), salt, and pepper.

3. Pour the dressing over the cabbage mixture and toss well to mix.

4. Allow the slaw to sit for at least 10 minutes to let the flavors meld together before serving.

5. If desired, garnish with chopped fresh parsley before serving.

Nutritional Information (per serving):

- **Total calories:** 50
- **Protein:** 1g
- **Fiber content:** 3g
- **Carbs:** 10g
- **Fats:** 2g

Roasted Tomato and Garlic Soup

Time to Prepare: 10 minutes
Cook Time: 40 minutes
Number of Servings: 4

List of Ingredients:

- 4 cups of ripe tomatoes, halved
- 1 whole head of garlic, cloves separated and peeled
- 1 medium onion, chopped
- 2 cups of low-sodium vegetable broth
- 1 tablespoon olive oil (optional; can be replaced with cooking spray for zero points)
- Salt and pepper, to taste
- 1 teaspoon of dried basil (or fresh basil, for garnish)

Instructions:

1. Preheat the oven to 400°F (200°C). Place the halved tomatoes and garlic cloves on a baking sheet. Drizzle with olive oil (if using) and season with salt and pepper.

2. Roast in the preheated oven for 25-30 minutes, or until the tomatoes are softened and slightly caramelized.

3. In a large pot, sauté the chopped onion over medium heat until translucent, about 5 minutes.

4. Add the roasted tomatoes and garlic to the pot, along with the vegetable broth. Bring to a boil, then reduce heat and simmer for 10 minutes.

5. Use an immersion blender to puree the soup until smooth (or carefully transfer to a blender in batches).

6. Adjust seasoning as needed. Serve hot, garnished with fresh basil if desired.

Nutritional Information (per serving):

- **Total calories:** 80
- **Protein:** 2g
- **Fiber content:** 3g
- **Carbs:** 15g
- **Fats:** 3g

Mushroom and Green Bean Stir-Fry

Time to Prepare: 10 minutes
Cook Time: 15 minutes
Number of Servings: 4

List of Ingredients:

- 2 cups of green beans, trimmed
- 2 cups of mushrooms, sliced (any variety)
- 1 medium onion, sliced
- 2 cloves garlic, minced
- 1 tablespoon low-sodium soy sauce
- 1 tablespoon fresh ginger, grated
- 1 teaspoon of sesame oil (optional; can be replaced with cooking spray for zero points)
- Salt and pepper, to taste
- Sesame seeds, for garnish (optional)

Instructions:

1. In a large skillet or wok, heat sesame oil (if using) over medium-high heat. Add the sliced onion and minced garlic, sautéing for 2-3 minutes until fragrant.

2. Add the sliced mushrooms and green beans to the skillet. Stir-fry for 5-7 minutes, or until the vegetables are tender-crisp.

3. Stir in the grated ginger and low-sodium soy sauce, cooking for an additional 2 minutes.

4. Season with salt and pepper to taste. Remove from heat.

5. Serve hot, garnished with sesame seeds if desired.

Nutritional Information (per serving):

- **Total calories:** 70
- **Protein:** 3g
- **Fiber content:** 4g
- **Carbs:** 13g
- **Fats:** 2g

Chicken and Spinach Wrap (using large lettuce leaves)

Time to Prepare: 10 minutes
Cook Time: 10 minutes
Number of Servings: 4

List of Ingredients:

- 2 cups of cooked chicken breast, shredded
- 2 cups of fresh spinach leaves
- 1/2 cup of diced tomatoes
- 1/4 cup of red onion, finely chopped
- 1/4 cup of low-fat Greek yogurt (for dressing)
- 1 tablespoon lemon juice
- Salt and pepper, to taste
- Large lettuce leaves (such as romaine or butter lettuce) for wrapping

Instructions:

1. In a bowl, mix the shredded chicken, fresh spinach, diced tomatoes, and red onion.
2. In a separate small bowl, mix the Greek yogurt, lemon juice, salt, and pepper to create a dressing.
3. Pour the dressing over the chicken and vegetable mixture, and toss until well coated.
4. Take a large lettuce leaf and fill it with a portion of the chicken and spinach mixture. Wrap it tightly.
5. Repeat with the remaining lettuce leaves and filling. Serve immediately.

Nutritional Information (per serving):

- **Total calories:** 150
- **Protein:** 25g
- **Fiber content:** 2g
- **Carbs:** 6g
- **Fats:** 3g

Spicy Lentil and Tomato Soup

Time to Prepare: 10 minutes
Cook Time: 30 minutes
Number of Servings: 6

List of Ingredients:

- 1 cup of dried lentils, rinsed
- 1 can (15 oz) diced tomatoes (no added sugar or salt)
- 1 medium onion, chopped
- 2 cloves garlic, minced
- 4 cups of vegetable broth (low sodium)
- 2 carrots, diced
- 2 celery stalks, diced
- 1 teaspoon of cumin
- 1 teaspoon of smoked paprika
- 1/2 teaspoon of red pepper flakes (adjust to taste)
- Salt and pepper, to taste
- Fresh cilantro or parsley for garnish (optional)

Instructions:

1. In a large pot, sauté the chopped onion and minced garlic over medium heat until translucent, about 5 minutes.
2. Add the diced carrots and celery, cooking for another 5 minutes until softened.
3. Stir in the rinsed lentils, diced tomatoes, vegetable broth, cumin, smoked paprika, and red pepper flakes.
4. Bring the mixture to a boil, then reduce heat to low. Cover and simmer for about 25 minutes, or until the lentils are tender.
5. Season with salt and pepper to taste. Serve hot, garnished with fresh cilantro or parsley if desired.

Nutritional Information (per serving):

- **Total calories:** 150
- **Protein:** 9g
- **Fiber content:** 6g
- **Carbs:** 27g
- **Fats:** 0g

CHAPTER 3: DINNER

Lemon Garlic Chicken with Roasted Veggies

Time to Prepare: 15 minutes
Cook Time: 35 minutes
Number of Servings: 4

List of Ingredients:

- 4 boneless, skinless chicken breasts
- 2 tablespoons olive oil
- 2 tablespoons lemon juice
- 4 cloves garlic, minced
- 1 teaspoon of dried oregano
- 1 teaspoon of paprika
- Salt and pepper, to taste
- 2 cups of broccoli florets
- 1 cup of bell peppers, sliced
- 1 cup of zucchini, sliced
- 1 cup of cherry tomatoes

Instructions:

1. Preheat the oven to 400°F (200°C).
2. In a small bowl, mix olive oil, lemon juice, minced garlic, oregano, paprika, salt, and pepper to create a marinade.
3. Place the chicken breasts in a large zip-top bag or bowl and pour the marinade over them. Let marinate for at least 15 minutes.
4. While the chicken is marinating, prepare the vegetables. In a large bowl, toss broccoli, bell peppers, zucchini, and cherry tomatoes with a drizzle of olive oil, salt, and pepper.
5. Spread the vegetables evenly on a baking sheet and place the marinated chicken breasts on top.
6. Bake for 25-30 minutes or until the chicken is cooked through and the vegetables are tender, stirring the vegetables halfway through.
7. Serve hot, garnished with fresh lemon slices if desired.

Nutritional Information (per serving):

- **Total calories:** 210
- **Protein:** 28g
- **Fiber content:** 4g
- **Carbs:** 10g
- **Fats:** 8g

Baked Tilapia with Citrus Salsa

Time to Prepare: 10 minutes
Cook Time: 20 minutes
Number of Servings: 4

List of Ingredients:

- 4 tilapia fillets

- 1 tablespoon olive oil

- 1 teaspoon of garlic powder

- 1 teaspoon of paprika

- Salt and pepper, to taste

- 1 cup of diced pineapple

- 1 cup of diced mango

- 1/2 cup of diced red onion

- 1/4 cup of fresh cilantro, chopped

- Juice of 1 lime

- Juice of 1 orange

Instructions:

1. Preheat the oven to 375°F (190°C).

2. Place the tilapia fillets on a baking sheet lined with parchment paper. Drizzle with olive oil and season with garlic powder, paprika, salt, and pepper.

3. Bake the tilapia for 15-20 minutes or until the fish flakes easily with a fork.

4. While the fish is baking, prepare the citrus salsa. In a bowl, mix diced pineapple, mango, red onion, cilantro, lime juice, and orange juice. Mix well.

5. Serve the baked tilapia topped with the citrus salsa.

Nutritional Information (per serving):

- **Total calories:** 180

- **Protein:** 22g

- **Fiber content:** 3g

- **Carbs:** 15g

- **Fats:** 7g

Zucchini Lasagna (using zucchini slices as "noodles")

Time to Prepare: 20 minutes
Cook Time: 30 minutes
Number of Servings: 6

List of Ingredients:

- 4 medium zucchini, sliced into thin strips
- 2 cups of marinara sauce (no added sugar)
- 1 cup of ricotta cheese (low-fat)
- 1 cup of shredded mozzarella cheese (part-skim)
- 1/2 cup of grated Parmesan cheese
- 1 egg
- 2 cups of fresh spinach
- 1 teaspoon of Italian seasoning
- Salt and pepper, to taste
- Cooking spray

Instructions:

1. Preheat the oven to 375°F (190°C). Lightly spray a 9x13-inch baking dish with cooking spray.

2. In a bowl, mix the ricotta cheese, egg, spinach, Italian seasoning, salt, and pepper until well mixed.

3. Spread a thin layer of marinara sauce on the bottom of the prepared baking dish. Layer half of the zucchini slices over the sauce.

4. Spread half of the ricotta mixture over the zucchini. Top with another layer of marinara sauce and half of the mozzarella cheese.

5. Repeat the layers with the remaining zucchini, ricotta mixture, marinara sauce, and finish with the remaining mozzarella and Parmesan cheese on top.

6. Cover with aluminum foil and bake for 20 minutes. Remove the foil and bake for an additional 10 minutes, or until the cheese is bubbly and golden.

7. Let it cool for a few minutes before slicing and serving.

Nutritional Information (per serving):

- **Total calories:** 190
- **Protein:** 14g
- **Fiber content:** 3g
- **Carbs:** 15g
- **Fats:** 9g

Stuffed Bell Peppers with Ground Turkey

Time to Prepare: 15 minutes
Cook Time: 30 minutes
Number of Servings: 4

List of Ingredients:

- 4 large bell peppers (any color)
- 1 pound lean ground turkey
- 1 cup of cooked brown rice (or cauliflower rice for a lower-carb option)
- 1 cup of diced tomatoes (canned, no added sugar)
- 1 small onion, chopped
- 2 cloves garlic, minced
- 1 teaspoon of Italian seasoning
- Salt and pepper, to taste
- 1/2 cup of shredded low-fat cheese (optional, for topping)
- Cooking spray

Instructions:

1. Preheat the oven to 375°F (190°C). Lightly spray a baking dish with cooking spray.
2. Cut the tops off the bell peppers and remove the seeds and membranes. Place the peppers upright in the prepared baking dish.
3. In a skillet over medium heat, sauté the onion and garlic until softened. Add the ground turkey and cook until browned.
4. Stir in the cooked brown rice, diced tomatoes, Italian seasoning, salt, and pepper. Cook for an additional 2-3 minutes until heated through.
5. Spoon the turkey mixture into each bell pepper, packing it down slightly. If using, sprinkle the shredded cheese on top of each stuffed pepper.
6. Cover the baking dish with foil and bake for 25 minutes. Remove the foil and bake for an additional 5 minutes until the peppers are tender.
7. Let cool for a few minutes before serving.

Nutritional Information (per serving):

- **Total calories:** 220
- **Protein:** 25g
- **Fiber content:** 4g
- **Carbs:** 18g
- **Fats:** 7g

Herb-Crusted Cod with Steamed Asparagus

Time to Prepare: 10 minutes
Cook Time: 20 minutes
Number of Servings: 4

List of Ingredients:

- 4 cod fillets (approximately 4 ounces each)
- 1 cup of fresh breadcrumbs (made from whole grain bread)
- 2 tablespoons fresh parsley, chopped
- 1 tablespoon fresh dill, chopped
- 1 teaspoon of garlic powder
- 1 teaspoon of onion powder
- Salt and pepper, to taste
- 1 tablespoon olive oil
- 1 pound fresh asparagus, trimmed
- Lemon wedges (for serving)

Instructions:

1. Preheat the oven to 400°F (200°C). Line a baking sheet with parchment paper.
2. In a bowl, mix the breadcrumbs, parsley, dill, garlic powder, onion powder, salt, and pepper. Mix well.
3. Drizzle the cod fillets with olive oil and season with additional salt and pepper. Press the breadcrumb mixture onto the top of each fillet.
4. Place the cod fillets on the prepared baking sheet and bake for 15-20 minutes, or until the fish flakes easily with a fork and the crust is golden.
5. While the cod is baking, bring a pot of water to a boil. Add the asparagus and steam for 3-5 minutes until tender but still bright green.
6. Serve the herb-crusted cod with steamed asparagus and lemon wedges on the side.

Nutritional Information (per serving):

- **Total calories:** 220
- **Protein:** 30g
- **Fiber content:** 5g
- **Carbs:** 15g
- **Fats:** 7g

Turkey and Veggie Stir-Fry

Time to Prepare: 10 minutes
Cook Time: 15 minutes
Number of Servings: 4

List of Ingredients:

- 1 pound lean ground turkey
- 2 cups of mixed vegetables (such as bell peppers, broccoli, and snap peas)
- 1 tablespoon low-sodium soy sauce
- 1 tablespoon fresh ginger, minced
- 2 cloves garlic, minced
- 1 tablespoon sesame oil
- Salt and pepper, to taste
- 2 green onions, chopped (for garnish)

Instructions:

1. In a large skillet or wok, heat sesame oil over medium-high heat.
2. Add minced garlic and ginger, and sauté for 1 minute until fragrant.
3. Add the ground turkey, breaking it up with a spoon. Cook until browned and cooked through, about 5-7 minutes.
4. Stir in the mixed vegetables and soy sauce. Cook for an additional 5-7 minutes until the vegetables are tender-crisp.
5. Season with salt and pepper to taste. Remove from heat.
6. Serve hot, garnished with chopped green onions.

Nutritional Information (per serving):

- **Total calories:** 220
- **Protein:** 28g
- **Fiber content:** 4g
- **Carbs:** 10g
- **Fats:** 10g

Cabbage and Carrot "Noodle" Pad Thai

Time to Prepare: 15 minutes
Cook Time: 10 minutes
Number of Servings: 4

List of Ingredients:

- 4 cups of green cabbage, thinly sliced
- 2 cups of carrots, julienned
- 1 cup of bell pepper, sliced
- 1 cup of green onions, chopped
- 2 tablespoons low-sodium soy sauce
- 1 tablespoon peanut butter (optional, for flavor)
- 2 cloves garlic, minced
- 1 tablespoon lime juice
- 1 tablespoon rice vinegar
- 1 teaspoon of fresh ginger, minced
- Crushed red pepper flakes (to taste)
- Fresh cilantro (for garnish)

Instructions:

1. In a large skillet or wok, heat a splash of water or cooking spray over medium heat.
2. Add minced garlic and ginger, and sauté for 1 minute until fragrant.
3. Add sliced cabbage, carrots, and bell pepper. Stir-fry for about 5-7 minutes until the vegetables are tender but still crisp.
4. In a small bowl, whisk together soy sauce, peanut butter (if using), lime juice, and rice vinegar.
5. Pour the sauce over the vegetables and stir well to mix. Cook for an additional 2-3 minutes.
6. Remove from heat and season with crushed red pepper flakes to taste. Garnish with chopped green onions and cilantro before serving.

Nutritional Information (per serving):

- **Total calories:** 70
- **Protein:** 2g
- **Fiber content:** 4g
- **Carbs:** 12g
- **Fats:** 3g

Eggplant and Tomato Bake

Time to Prepare: 15 minutes
Cook Time: 40 minutes
Number of Servings: 4

List of Ingredients:

- 2 medium eggplants, sliced

- 4 cups of tomatoes, diced (canned or fresh)

- 1 medium onion, chopped

- 3 cloves garlic, minced

- 1 teaspoon of dried oregano

- 1 teaspoon of dried basil

- 1 teaspoon of salt

- 1/2 teaspoon of black pepper

- Cooking spray or a splash of vegetable broth

Instructions:

1. Preheat the oven to 375°F (190°C).

2. In a large skillet, spray with cooking spray or add a splash of vegetable broth. Sauté the chopped onion and minced garlic over medium heat until softened, about 5 minutes.

3. In a baking dish, layer half of the sliced eggplant at the bottom. Top with half of the diced tomatoes, half of the sautéed onion and garlic mixture, and sprinkle with half of the oregano, basil, salt, and pepper. Repeat the layers with the remaining ingredients.

4. Cover the dish with aluminum foil and bake for 30 minutes.

5. Remove the foil and bake for an additional 10 minutes, or until the eggplant is tender and the top is slightly golden.

6. Allow to cool for a few minutes before serving.

Nutritional Information (per serving):

- **Total calories:** 80

- **Protein:** 3g

- **Fiber content:** 5g

- **Carbs:** 15g

- **Fats:** 1g

Lemon Herb Shrimp with Broccoli

Time to Prepare: 10 minutes
Cook Time: 10 minutes
Number of Servings: 4

List of Ingredients:

- 1 pound shrimp, peeled and deveined
- 4 cups of broccoli florets
- 2 tablespoons lemon juice
- 2 teaspoons of olive oil
- 3 cloves garlic, minced
- 1 teaspoon of dried oregano
- 1 teaspoon of dried parsley
- Salt and pepper to taste
- Cooking spray or a splash of vegetable broth

Instructions:

1. In a large skillet, spray with cooking spray or add a splash of vegetable broth over medium heat.
2. Add the minced garlic and sauté for 1 minute until fragrant.
3. Add the broccoli florets to the skillet and sauté for 3-4 minutes until tender-crisp.
4. Push the broccoli to the side of the skillet and add the shrimp.
5. Drizzle with olive oil, lemon juice, oregano, parsley, salt, and pepper. Cook for 3-5 minutes, stirring occasionally, until the shrimp are pink and opaque.
6. Serve warm, garnished with additional lemon wedges if desired.

Nutritional Information (per serving):

- **Total calories:** 120
- **Protein:** 23g
- **Fiber content:** 3g
- **Carbs:** 6g
- **Fats:** 2g

Chili with Lean Ground Chicken

Time to Prepare: 10 minutes
Cook Time: 30 minutes
Number of Servings: 6

List of Ingredients:

- 1 pound lean ground chicken

- 1 medium onion, chopped

- 2 cloves garlic, minced

- 1 bell pepper, chopped

- 2 cans (15 ounces each) diced tomatoes (no salt added)

- 1 can (15 ounces) black beans, rinsed and drained

- 1 can (15 ounces) kidney beans, rinsed and drained

- 2 tablespoons chili powder

- 1 teaspoon of cumin

- 1 teaspoon of paprika

- Salt and pepper to taste

- 1 cup of corn (fresh or frozen)

- 1 cup of low-sodium chicken broth

Instructions:

1. In a large pot, spray with cooking spray and sauté the onion, garlic, and bell pepper over medium heat until softened, about 5 minutes.

2. Add the ground chicken to the pot and cook until browned, breaking it up as it cooks.

3. Stir in the diced tomatoes, black beans, kidney beans, chili powder, cumin, paprika, salt, pepper, corn, and chicken broth.

4. Bring to a boil, then reduce the heat and simmer for about 20 minutes, stirring occasionally.

5. Adjust seasoning to taste before serving.

Nutritional Information (per serving):

- **Total calories:** 190

- **Protein:** 22g

- **Fiber content:** 7g

- **Carbs:** 23g

- **Fats:** 3g

Baked Spaghetti Squash with Marinara Sauce

Time to Prepare: 10 minutes
Cook Time: 45 minutes
Number of Servings: 4

List of Ingredients:

- 1 medium spaghetti squash
- 2 cups of marinara sauce (no sugar added)
- 1 teaspoon of olive oil
- 1 teaspoon of garlic powder
- 1 teaspoon of Italian seasoning
- Salt and pepper to taste
- Fresh basil for garnish (optional)

Instructions:

1. Preheat the oven to 400°F (200°C).
2. Cut the spaghetti squash in half lengthwise and scoop out the seeds.
3. Brush the inside of each half with olive oil and sprinkle with garlic powder, Italian seasoning, salt, and pepper.
4. Place the squash cut-side down on a baking sheet and bake for 30-35 minutes, or until tender.
5. Once baked, let the squash cool for a few minutes. Then, using a fork, scrape the inside to create spaghetti-like strands.
6. In a saucepan, heat the marinara sauce over medium heat until warmed through.
7. Serve the spaghetti squash topped with marinara sauce and garnish with fresh basil if desired.

Nutritional Information (per serving):

- **Total calories:** 130
- **Protein:** 4g
- **Fiber content:** 5g
- **Carbs:** 24g
- **Fats:** 3g

Cauliflower Fried Rice with Shrimp

Time to Prepare: 10 minutes
Cook Time: 15 minutes
Number of Servings: 4

List of Ingredients:

- 4 cups of riced cauliflower (fresh or frozen)
- 1 cup of cooked shrimp (peeled and deveined)
- 1 cup of mixed vegetables (carrots, peas, bell peppers)
- 2 cloves garlic (minced)
- 2 green onions (sliced)
- 2 tablespoons low-sodium soy sauce
- 1 tablespoon sesame oil (optional)
- Salt and pepper to taste
- Cooking spray or a small amount of water for sautéing

Instructions:

1. Heat a large skillet or wok over medium heat and coat with cooking spray or a small amount of water.
2. Add the minced garlic and cook for about 1 minute until fragrant.
3. Stir in the mixed vegetables and cook for 3-4 minutes until they are tender.
4. Add the riced cauliflower to the skillet and stir-fry for about 5 minutes until heated through.
5. Add the cooked shrimp, soy sauce, and sesame oil (if using). Stir well to mix and heat for an additional 2-3 minutes.
6. Season with salt and pepper to taste, and stir in the sliced green onions before serving.

Nutritional Information (per serving):

- **Total calories:** 150
- **Protein:** 14g
- **Fiber content:** 4g
- **Carbs:** 12g
- **Fats:** 5g

Garlicky Spinach and Mushroom Sauté with Chicken

Time to Prepare: 10 minutes
Cook Time: 15 minutes
Number of Servings: 4

List of Ingredients:

- 1 pound boneless, skinless chicken breast (sliced into strips)
- 4 cups of fresh spinach
- 8 ounces mushrooms (sliced)
- 4 cloves garlic (minced)
- 1 tablespoon olive oil
- 1 teaspoon of dried oregano
- Salt and pepper to taste
- Cooking spray or a small amount of water for sautéing

Instructions:

1. Heat a large skillet over medium heat and spray with cooking spray or add a small amount of water.
2. Add the olive oil and minced garlic to the skillet, cooking for about 1 minute until fragrant.
3. Add the sliced chicken breast and cook until browned and cooked through, about 5-7 minutes. Season with salt, pepper, and oregano.
4. Stir in the sliced mushrooms and cook for another 3-4 minutes until softened.
5. Add the fresh spinach and cook until wilted, about 2 minutes. Stir well to mix and serve immediately.

Nutritional Information (per serving):

- **Total calories:** 180
- **Protein:** 30g
- **Fiber content:** 3g
- **Carbs:** 6g
- **Fats:** 5g

Roasted Tomato and Eggplant Stew

Time to Prepare: 15 minutes
Cook Time: 45 minutes
Number of Servings: 4

List of Ingredients:

- 2 medium eggplants (cubed)
- 4 cups of cherry tomatoes (halved)
- 1 medium onion (diced)
- 4 cloves garlic (minced)
- 1 tablespoon olive oil
- 1 teaspoon of dried basil
- 1 teaspoon of dried oregano
- Salt and pepper to taste
- Fresh basil for garnish (optional)

Instructions:

1. Preheat the oven to 400°F (200°C).
2. In a large mixing bowl, mix the cubed eggplant, halved cherry tomatoes, diced onion, and minced garlic.
3. Drizzle with olive oil and sprinkle with dried basil, oregano, salt, and pepper. Toss to coat evenly.
4. Spread the mixture onto a large baking sheet in a single layer.
5. Roast in the oven for 30-35 minutes, stirring halfway through, until the vegetables are tender and slightly caramelized.
6. Remove from the oven and let cool slightly before serving. Garnish with fresh basil if desired.

Nutritional Information (per serving):

- **Total calories:** 120
- **Protein:** 3g
- **Fiber content:** 5g
- **Carbs:** 18g
- **Fats:** 5g

Grilled Salmon with Mango Salsa

Time to Prepare: 15 minutes
Cook Time: 10 minutes
Number of Servings: 4

List of Ingredients:

- 4 salmon fillets (6 oz each)
- 1 ripe mango (diced)
- 1 red bell pepper (diced)
- 1/4 red onion (finely chopped)
- 1 jalapeño (seeded and minced)
- Juice of 1 lime
- 1 tablespoon fresh cilantro (chopped)
- Salt and pepper to taste
- Cooking spray

Instructions:

1. Preheat the grill to medium-high heat and spray with cooking spray.
2. Season the salmon fillets with salt and pepper on both sides.
3. Grill the salmon for about 4-5 minutes per side or until cooked through and flaky.
4. While the salmon is grilling, prepare the mango salsa by combining diced mango, red bell pepper, red onion, jalapeño, lime juice, cilantro, salt, and pepper in a bowl. Mix well.
5. Remove the salmon from the grill and serve topped with mango salsa.

Nutritional Information (per serving):

- **Total calories:** 280
- **Protein:** 26g
- **Fiber content:** 2g
- **Carbs:** 12g
- **Fats:** 15g

Mexican Cauliflower Rice with Black Beans

Time to Prepare: 10 minutes
Cook Time: 15 minutes
Number of Servings: 4

List of Ingredients:

- 1 head of cauliflower (riced, about 4 cups of)
- 1 can (15 oz) black beans (rinsed and drained)
- 1 red bell pepper (diced)
- 1 green bell pepper (diced)
- 1 small onion (diced)
- 2 cloves garlic (minced)
- 1 teaspoon of chili powder
- 1 teaspoon of cumin
- 1/2 teaspoon of paprika
- Salt and pepper to taste
- 1/2 cup of chopped fresh cilantro
- Juice of 1 lime
- Cooking spray

Instructions:

1. Heat a large skillet over medium heat and spray with cooking spray.
2. Add the onion, red bell pepper, green bell pepper, and garlic. Sauté for 3-4 minutes until softened.
3. Stir in the riced cauliflower, black beans, chili powder, cumin, paprika, salt, and pepper.
4. Cook for 5-7 minutes, stirring occasionally, until the cauliflower is tender.
5. Remove from heat, stir in lime juice and cilantro.
6. Serve hot.

Nutritional Information (per serving):

- **Total calories:** 120
- **Protein:** 6g
- **Fiber content:** 7g
- **Carbs:** 20g
- **Fats:** 1g

Dijon Mustard Chicken with Green Beans

Time to Prepare: 10 minutes
Cook Time: 20 minutes
Number of Servings: 4

List of Ingredients:

- 4 boneless, skinless chicken breasts
- 2 tablespoons Dijon mustard
- 1 teaspoon of garlic powder
- Salt and pepper to taste
- 1 lb green beans (trimmed)
- Juice of 1 lemon
- Cooking spray

Instructions:

1. Preheat a large skillet over medium heat and spray with cooking spray.
2. Season chicken breasts with salt, pepper, and garlic powder.
3. Add chicken breasts to the skillet and cook for 5-6 minutes on each side, until fully cooked.
4. Brush each chicken breast with Dijon mustard during the last 2 minutes of cooking.
5. Meanwhile, steam or sauté green beans for 5-7 minutes until tender-crisp.
6. Drizzle lemon juice over green beans before serving.
7. Serve chicken alongside green beans.

Nutritional Information (per serving):

- **Total calories:** 140
- **Protein:** 26g
- **Fiber content:** 4g
- **Carbs:** 5g
- **Fats:** 2g

Sweet and Spicy Baked Chicken Thighs

Time to Prepare: 10 minutes
Cook Time: 25 minutes
Number of Servings: 4

List of Ingredients:

- 8 skinless, boneless chicken thighs
- 1 teaspoon of garlic powder
- 1 teaspoon of paprika
- 1 teaspoon of chili powder
- 1 teaspoon of ground cumin
- 1/2 teaspoon of salt
- 1/2 teaspoon of black pepper
- 1 tablespoon lemon juice
- Cooking spray

Instructions:

1. Preheat oven to 400°F (200°C). Lightly spray a baking dish with cooking spray.
2. In a small bowl, mix garlic powder, paprika, chili powder, ground cumin, salt, and black pepper.
3. Rub spice mixture evenly over both sides of the chicken thighs.
4. Place chicken in the prepared baking dish and drizzle with lemon juice.
5. Bake for 20-25 minutes or until the chicken reaches an internal temperature of 165°F (74°C).
6. Serve hot.

Nutritional Information (per serving):

- **Total calories:** 150
- **Protein:** 24g
- **Fiber content:** 0g
- **Carbs:** 1g
- **Fats:** 4g

CHAPTER 4: SNACKS

Air-Fried Zucchini Chips

Time to Prepare: 10 minutes
Cook Time: 15 minutes
Number of Servings: 4

List of Ingredients:

- 2 medium zucchinis, thinly sliced
- 1 teaspoon of garlic powder
- 1 teaspoon of onion powder
- 1/2 teaspoon of salt
- 1/2 teaspoon of black pepper
- Cooking spray

Instructions:

1. Preheat the air fryer to 400°F (200°C).
2. In a bowl, toss zucchini slices with garlic powder, onion powder, salt, and black pepper.
3. Lightly coat the air fryer basket with cooking spray.
4. Place seasoned zucchini slices in a single layer in the air fryer basket.
5. Cook for 10-15 minutes, shaking the basket halfway through, until zucchini chips are crispy and golden.
6. Serve immediately.

Nutritional Information (per serving):

- **Total calories:** 35
- **Protein:** 2g
- **Fiber content:** 2g
- **Carbs:** 7g
- **Fats:** 0g

Spiced Roasted Chickpeas

Time to Prepare: 5 minutes
Cook Time: 30 minutes
Number of Servings: 4

List of Ingredients:

- 1 can (15 oz) chickpeas, drained and rinsed
- 1 teaspoon of paprika
- 1 teaspoon of cumin
- 1/2 teaspoon of garlic powder
- 1/2 teaspoon of salt
- Cooking spray

Instructions:

1. Preheat oven to 400°F (200°C).
2. Pat the chickpeas dry with a paper towel.
3. In a bowl, toss chickpeas with paprika, cumin, garlic powder, and salt.
4. Lightly coat a baking sheet with cooking spray and spread chickpeas in a single layer.
5. Roast for 25-30 minutes, shaking the pan halfway through, until chickpeas are crispy.
6. Let cool slightly before serving.

Nutritional Information (per serving):

- **Total calories:** 90
- **Protein:** 5g
- **Fiber content:** 4g
- **Carbs:** 14g
- **Fats:** 1g

Baked Apple Chips

Time to Prepare: 10 minutes
Cook Time: 2 hours
Number of Servings: 4

List of Ingredients:

- 2 large apples, thinly sliced

- 1/2 teaspoon of ground cinnamon

Instructions:

1. Preheat oven to 200°F (95°C).

2. Arrange apple slices in a single layer on a baking sheet lined with parchment paper.

3. Sprinkle with cinnamon.

4. Bake for 2 hours, turning slices halfway through, until apples are crisp.

5. Let cool completely before serving.

Nutritional Information (per serving):

- **Total calories:** 50

- **Protein:** 0g

- **Fiber content:** 3g

- **Carbs:** 13g

- **Fats:** 0g

Cucumber Slices with Salsa

Time to Prepare: 10 minutes
Cook Time: 0 minutes
Number of Servings: 4

List of Ingredients:

- 2 large cucumbers, thinly sliced

- 1 cup of fresh salsa (diced tomatoes, onion, jalapeño, cilantro, lime juice, salt)

Instructions:

1. Arrange cucumber slices on a serving platter.

2. Top each slice with a spoonful of fresh salsa.

3. Serve immediately or refrigerate until ready to serve.

Nutritional Information (per serving):

- **Total calories:** 20

- **Protein:** 1g

- **Fiber content:** 2g

- **Carbs:** 4g

- **Fats:** 0g

Roasted Red Pepper Hummus with Veggie Sticks

Time to Prepare: 10 minutes
Cook Time: 0 minutes
Number of Servings: 4

List of Ingredients:

- 1 cup of canned chickpeas, drained and rinsed

- 1 roasted red bell pepper, chopped

- 1 clove garlic, minced

- 2 tablespoons lemon juice

- 1 teaspoon of ground cumin

- Salt and pepper to taste

- 1/4 cup of water (as needed for consistency)

- Assorted veggie sticks (carrots, celery, cucumber)

Instructions:

1. In a food processor, mix chickpeas, roasted red bell pepper, garlic, lemon juice, cumin, salt, and pepper.

2. Blend until smooth, adding water as needed to reach desired consistency.

3. Serve with assorted veggie sticks for dipping.

Nutritional Information (per serving):

- **Total calories:** 60

- **Protein:** 3g

- **Fiber content:** 4g

- **Carbs:** 11g

- **Fats:** 0g

Mixed Berry Popsicles (using plain Greek yogurt)

Time to Prepare: 10 minutes
Cook Time: 0 minutes (plus 4 hours freezing time)
Number of Servings: 6

List of Ingredients:

- 1 cup of plain non-fat Greek yogurt
- 1 cup of mixed berries (strawberries, blueberries, raspberries)
- 1 teaspoon of vanilla extract
- 1-2 tablespoons water (if needed for blending)

Instructions:

1. In a blender, mix the Greek yogurt, mixed berries, and vanilla extract. Blend until smooth.
2. Add a little water if the mixture is too thick to blend.
3. Pour the mixture into popsicle molds.
4. Freeze for at least 4 hours or until solid.
5. Remove from molds and enjoy.

Nutritional Information (per serving):

- **Total calories:** 30
- **Protein:** 4g
- **Fiber content:** 1g
- **Carbs:** 5g
- **Fats:** 0g

Hard-Boiled Eggs with Everything Bagel Seasoning

Time to Prepare: 5 minutes
Cook Time: 10 minutes
Number of Servings: 4

List of Ingredients:

- 4 large eggs
- 1 tablespoon Everything Bagel seasoning

Instructions:

1. Place eggs in a saucepan and cover with water.
2. Bring to a boil, then reduce heat and simmer for 9-10 minutes.
3. Remove eggs and place in an ice bath for a few minutes to cool.
4. Peel the eggs and sprinkle with Everything Bagel seasoning before serving.

Nutritional Information (per serving):

- **Total calories:** 70
- **Protein:** 6g
- **Fiber content:** 0g
- **Carbs:** 1g
- **Fats:** 5g

Watermelon and Mint Salad

Time to Prepare: 10 minutes
Cook Time: 0 minutes
Number of Servings: 4

List of Ingredients:

- 4 cups of watermelon, cubed
- 1/4 cup of fresh mint leaves, chopped
- 1 tablespoon lime juice
- Salt, to taste (optional)

Instructions:

1. In a large bowl, mix the cubed watermelon and chopped mint leaves.
2. Drizzle lime juice over the salad and gently toss to mix.
3. Season with a pinch of salt if desired.
4. Serve immediately or refrigerate for up to 30 minutes before serving to enhance flavors.

Nutritional Information (per serving):

- **Total calories:** 50
- **Protein:** 1g
- **Fiber content:** 1g
- **Carbs:** 13g
- **Fats:** 0g

Mango and Pineapple Salsa with Bell Pepper Slices

Time to Prepare: 15 minutes
Cook Time: 0 minutes
Number of Servings: 4

List of Ingredients:

- 1 ripe mango, diced
- 1 cup of pineapple, diced
- 1/2 red bell pepper, diced
- 1/2 green bell pepper, diced
- 1/4 cup of red onion, finely chopped
- 1 jalapeño, seeds removed and minced (optional)
- 2 tablespoons lime juice
- Salt and pepper, to taste
- 1 large bell pepper, sliced (for serving)

Instructions:

1. In a medium bowl, mix the diced mango, pineapple, red bell pepper, green bell pepper, red onion, and jalapeño.
2. Drizzle lime juice over the mixture and season with salt and pepper to taste.
3. Gently toss to mix all ingredients.
4. Serve salsa with sliced bell peppers as dippers.

Nutritional Information (per serving):

- **Total calories:** 60
- **Protein:** 1g
- **Fiber content:** 2g
- **Carbs:** 15g
- **Fats:** 0g

Cucumber Roll-Ups with Turkey Slices

Time to Prepare: 10 minutes
Cook Time: 0 minutes
Number of Servings: 4

List of Ingredients:

- 1 large cucumber, thinly sliced into long strips
- 8 slices of deli turkey breast (low-sodium)
- 1/2 cup of cream cheese (light or reduced-fat)
- 1 tablespoon fresh dill, chopped (or 1 teaspoon of dried dill)
- Salt and pepper, to taste

Instructions:

1. In a small bowl, mix cream cheese with fresh dill, salt, and pepper until well mixed.
2. Spread a thin layer of the cream cheese mixture onto each turkey slice.
3. Place a cucumber strip at one end of the turkey slice and roll it up tightly.
4. Secure with a toothpick if necessary and repeat with the remaining ingredients.
5. Arrange the roll-ups on a serving platter and enjoy.

Nutritional Information (per serving):

- **Total calories:** 80
- **Protein:** 10g
- **Fiber content:** 1g
- **Carbs:** 2g
- **Fats:** 4g

Tomato Basil Bites

Time to Prepare: 10 minutes
Cook Time: 0 minutes
Number of Servings: 4

List of Ingredients:

- 12 cherry tomatoes, halved
- 1 cup of fresh basil leaves
- 4 ounces fresh mozzarella cheese, cubed (light or part-skim)
- 1 tablespoon balsamic vinegar
- Salt and pepper, to taste

Instructions:

1. In a bowl, mix cherry tomatoes, mozzarella cubes, and fresh basil leaves.
2. Drizzle with balsamic vinegar and season with salt and pepper.
3. Gently toss the mixture until evenly coated.
4. Serve immediately as bite-sized appetizers or refrigerate for up to 30 minutes before serving.

Nutritional Information (per serving):

- **Total calories:** 60
- **Protein:** 4g
- **Fiber content:** 1g
- **Carbs:** 4g
- **Fats:** 3g

Jicama Sticks with Lime and Chili Powder

Time to Prepare: 10 minutes
Cook Time: 0 minutes
Number of Servings: 4

List of Ingredients:

- 1 medium jicama, peeled and cut into sticks
- 1 lime, juiced
- 1 teaspoon of chili powder
- Salt, to taste

Instructions:

1. In a large bowl, mix the jicama sticks and lime juice.
2. Sprinkle with chili powder and salt.
3. Toss until the jicama is evenly coated with the lime juice and seasoning.
4. Serve immediately or chill in the refrigerator for 10 minutes before serving.

Nutritional Information (per serving):

- **Total calories:** 50
- **Protein:** 1g
- **Fiber content:** 5g
- **Carbs:** 12g
- **Fats:** 0g

Bell Pepper Nachos

Time to Prepare: 10 minutes
Cook Time: 0 minutes
Number of Servings: 4

List of Ingredients:

- 2 large bell peppers (any color), cut into strips
- 1 cup of salsa
- 1/2 cup of shredded reduced-fat cheese (optional for a zero point option)
- 1/4 cup of sliced black olives (optional)
- 1/4 cup of chopped green onions (optional)

Instructions:

1. Arrange the bell pepper strips on a serving platter to serve as "nacho chips."
2. Top with salsa, spreading it evenly over the pepper strips.
3. If using, sprinkle the reduced-fat cheese and add black olives on top.
4. Garnish with chopped green onions if desired.
5. Serve immediately as a fresh, crunchy snack.

Nutritional Information (per serving):

- **Total calories:** 40 | **Protein:** 1g
- **Fiber content:** 3g
- **Carbs:** 8g | **Fats:** 0g

Roasted Pumpkin Seeds

Time to Prepare: 10 minutes
Cook Time: 20 minutes
Number of Servings: 4

List of Ingredients:

- 1 cup of raw pumpkin seeds (pepitas)
- 1 teaspoon of olive oil (optional for zero points)
- 1 teaspoon of salt
- 1/2 teaspoon of garlic powder (optional)
- 1/2 teaspoon of paprika (optional)

Instructions:

1. Preheat the oven to 350°F (175°C).
2. Rinse the pumpkin seeds under cold water to remove any pulp. Pat dry with a paper towel.
3. In a bowl, mix the pumpkin seeds, olive oil (if using), salt, garlic powder, and paprika. Mix well to coat the seeds evenly.
4. Spread the seasoned pumpkin seeds in a single layer on a baking sheet.
5. Roast in the preheated oven for 15-20 minutes, stirring occasionally, until the seeds are golden brown and crunchy.
6. Remove from the oven and let cool before serving.

Nutritional Information (per serving):

- **Total calories:** 120
- **Protein:** 6g
- **Fiber content:** 2g
- **Carbs:** 4g
- **Fats:** 10g

Grilled Pineapple Rings with Cinnamon

Time to Prepare: 5 minutes
Cook Time: 10 minutes
Number of Servings: 4

List of Ingredients:

- 1 fresh pineapple, peeled and sliced into rings
- 1 teaspoon of ground cinnamon
- 1 teaspoon of honey (optional for zero points)
- Cooking spray (optional for grilling)

Instructions:

1. Preheat the grill or grill pan over medium heat.
2. Lightly spray the grill with cooking spray if desired.
3. Place the pineapple rings on the grill and sprinkle with cinnamon.
4. Grill for about 5 minutes on each side or until the pineapple is heated through and has grill marks.
5. Remove from the grill and, if using, drizzle with honey before serving.

Nutritional Information (per serving):

- **Total calories:** 50
- **Protein:** 0g
- **Fiber content:** 1g
- **Carbs:** 13g
- **Fats:** 0g

Carrot and Celery Sticks with Fat-Free Greek Yogurt Dip

Time to Prepare: 10 minutes
Cook Time: 0 minutes
Number of Servings: 4

List of Ingredients:

- 4 large carrots, cut into sticks
- 4 celery stalks, cut into sticks
- 1 cup of fat-free Greek yogurt
- 1 teaspoon of garlic powder
- 1 teaspoon of onion powder
- 1 teaspoon of dried dill
- Salt and pepper to taste

Instructions:

1. In a bowl, mix the fat-free Greek yogurt, garlic powder, onion powder, dill, salt, and pepper. Mix until well blended.
2. Arrange the carrot and celery sticks on a serving platter.
3. Serve the veggie sticks with the yogurt dip.

Nutritional Information (per serving):

- **Total calories:** 35
- **Protein:** 4g
- **Fiber content:** 2g
- **Carbs:** 6g
- **Fats:** 0g

Baked Kale Chips

Time to Prepare: 10 minutes
Cook Time: 20 minutes
Number of Servings: 4

List of Ingredients:

- 1 bunch kale, washed and dried
- 1 tablespoon olive oil
- 1 teaspoon of garlic powder
- 1 teaspoon of onion powder
- Salt to taste

Instructions:

1. Preheat the oven to 350°F (175°C).
2. Remove the kale leaves from the stems and tear them into bite-sized pieces.
3. In a large bowl, toss the kale with olive oil, garlic powder, onion powder, and salt until evenly coated.
4. Spread the kale in a single layer on a baking sheet.
5. Bake for 15-20 minutes, or until the edges are crisp but not burnt.
6. Remove from the oven and let cool before serving.

Nutritional Information (per serving):

- **Total calories:** 50
- **Protein:** 3g
- **Fiber content:** 2g
- **Carbs:** 7g
- **Fats:** 2g

Frozen Banana Bites

Time to Prepare: 10 minutes
Cook Time: 0 minutes
Number of Servings: 4

List of Ingredients:

- 2 ripe bananas, sliced

Instructions:

1. Line a baking sheet with parchment paper.

2. Arrange the banana slices in a single layer on the baking sheet.

3. Place the baking sheet in the freezer for about 1-2 hours, or until the banana slices are completely frozen.

4. Once frozen, transfer the banana bites to an airtight container or freezer bag for storage.

5. Serve frozen as a refreshing snack.

Nutritional Information (per serving):

- **Total calories:** 90
- **Protein:** 1g
- **Fiber content:** 2g
- **Carbs:** 23g
- **Fats:** 0g

Spicy Pickled Veggies

Time to Prepare: 15 minutes
Cook Time: 0 minutes
Number of Servings: 6

List of Ingredients:

- 1 cup of cucumber, sliced
- 1 cup of carrots, sliced
- 1 cup of bell peppers, sliced
- 1 cup of red onion, thinly sliced
- 1 cup of white vinegar
- 1 cup of water
- 2 tablespoons salt
- 1 tablespoon sugar (optional, adjust to taste)
- 1 teaspoon of red pepper flakes
- 1 teaspoon of garlic powder
- 1 teaspoon of mustard seeds

Instructions:

1. In a large bowl, mix the sliced cucumbers, carrots, bell peppers, and red onion.

2. In a separate bowl, mix the vinegar, water, salt, sugar, red pepper flakes, garlic powder, and mustard seeds until well mixed.

3. Pour the vinegar mixture over the vegetables, ensuring they are fully submerged.

4. Let the mixture sit for at least 1 hour at room temperature, or refrigerate for at least 2 hours to enhance the flavors.

5. Store the pickled veggies in an airtight container in the refrigerator for up to 2 weeks.

Nutritional Information (per serving):

- **Total calories:** 20
- **Protein:** 0g
- **Fiber content:** 1g
- **Carbs:** 4g
- **Fats:** 0g

Berry and Melon Skewers

Time to Prepare: 10 minutes
Cook Time: 0 minutes
Number of Servings: 4

List of Ingredients:

- 1 cup of strawberries, hulled and halved
- 1 cup of blueberries
- 1 cup of cantaloupe, cubed
- 1 cup of honeydew melon, cubed
- 1 tablespoon fresh mint, chopped (optional)
- 1 tablespoon lime juice

Instructions:

1. In a bowl, mix the strawberries, blueberries, cantaloupe, and honeydew.

2. Drizzle the lime juice over the fruit and gently toss to coat.

3. Thread the fruit onto skewers, alternating between the different types of fruit.

4. If desired, sprinkle with fresh mint before serving.

5. Serve immediately or refrigerate until ready to serve.

Nutritional Information (per serving):

- **Total calories:** 50
- **Protein:** 1g
- **Fiber content:** 2g
- **Carbs:** 12g
- **Fats:** 0g

CHAPTER 5: DESSERTS

Mixed Berry Compote

Time to Prepare: 5 minutes
Cook Time: 15 minutes
Number of Servings: 4

List of Ingredients:

- 2 cups of mixed berries (strawberries, blueberries, raspberries)
- 1/4 cup of water
- 1 tablespoon lemon juice
- 1 tablespoon honey or sugar substitute (optional)

Instructions:

1. In a saucepan, mix the mixed berries, water, and lemon juice.
2. Bring to a boil over medium heat, then reduce the heat and let simmer for about 10-15 minutes, stirring occasionally, until the berries are soft and the mixture has thickened slightly.
3. If desired, stir in honey or sugar substitute during the last few minutes of cooking for added sweetness.
4. Remove from heat and allow to cool slightly before serving.
5. Serve warm or chilled over yogurt, oatmeal, or enjoy on its own.

Nutritional Information (per serving):

- **Total calories:** 40
- **Protein:** 1g
- **Fiber content:** 3g
- **Carbs:** 10g
- **Fats:** 0g

Grilled Pineapple with Cinnamon

Time to Prepare: 5 minutes
Cook Time: 10 minutes
Number of Servings: 4

List of Ingredients:

- 1 medium pineapple, peeled and sliced into rings
- 1 teaspoon of ground cinnamon
- 1 tablespoon honey or sugar substitute (optional)

Instructions:

1. Preheat the grill to medium heat.
2. If desired, brush the pineapple rings lightly with honey or sugar substitute for added sweetness.
3. Sprinkle cinnamon evenly over both sides of the pineapple rings.
4. Place the pineapple rings on the grill and cook for about 4-5 minutes on each side, until grill marks appear and the pineapple is heated through.
5. Remove from the grill and serve warm.

Nutritional Information (per serving):

- **Total calories:** 50
- **Protein:** 1g
- **Fiber content:** 1g
- **Carbs:** 13g
- **Fats:** 0g

Frozen Banana Pops

Time to Prepare: 10 minutes
Cook Time: 0 minutes
Number of Servings: 4

List of Ingredients:

- 2 ripe bananas

- 1 cup of plain Greek yogurt

- 1 tablespoon honey or sugar substitute (optional)

- 1 teaspoon of vanilla extract (optional)

- Popsicle sticks

Instructions:

1. Peel the bananas and cut them in half. Insert a popsicle stick into the cut end of each banana half.

2. In a bowl, mix the Greek yogurt, honey or sugar substitute, and vanilla extract until smooth.

3. Dip each banana half into the yogurt mixture, ensuring it is well-coated.

4. Place the yogurt-coated bananas on a parchment-lined baking sheet.

5. Freeze the banana pops for at least 2 hours, or until firm.

6. Once frozen, remove from the freezer and enjoy!

Nutritional Information (per serving):

- **Total calories:** 90

- **Protein:** 4g

- **Fiber content:** 1g

- **Carbs:** 16g

- **Fats:** 0g

Baked Pears with Cinnamon and Nutmeg

Time to Prepare: 10 minutes
Cook Time: 25 minutes
Number of Servings: 4

List of Ingredients:

- 4 ripe pears, halved and cored

- 1 teaspoon of ground cinnamon

- 1/2 teaspoon of ground nutmeg

- 2 tablespoons honey or sugar substitute (optional)

- 1 cup of water

- Cooking spray (optional)

Instructions:

1. Preheat the oven to 350°F (175°C).

2. Place the pear halves in a baking dish, cut side up.

3. In a small bowl, mix the cinnamon and nutmeg together. Sprinkle the mixture over the pears.

4. If using, drizzle the honey or sugar substitute over the pears.

5. Pour the water into the bottom of the baking dish to create steam while baking.

6. Cover the dish with foil and bake for 20 minutes.

7. Remove the foil and bake for an additional 5 minutes, or until the pears are tender and slightly caramelized.

8. Serve warm, drizzled with the pan juices if desired.

Nutritional Information (per serving):

- **Total calories:** 90

- **Protein:** 1g

- **Fiber content:** 3g

- **Carbs:** 23g

- **Fats:** 0g

Strawberry Mango Sorbet

Time to Prepare: 10 minutes
Cook Time: 0 minutes
Number of Servings: 4

List of Ingredients:

- 2 cups of frozen strawberries

- 2 cups of frozen mango chunks

- 1 tablespoon lime juice

- 1-2 tablespoons honey or agave syrup (optional, adjust to taste)

- 1/2 cup of water (as needed for blending)

Instructions:

1. In a blender or food processor, mix the frozen strawberries, frozen mango, lime juice, and honey or agave syrup (if using).

2. Blend until smooth, adding water as needed to help blend the mixture into a sorbet consistency.

3. Taste and adjust sweetness if necessary by adding more honey or agave syrup.

4. Transfer the sorbet to a container and freeze for at least 1 hour to firm up if it is too soft.

5. Scoop and serve immediately. Store any leftovers in the freezer.

Nutritional Information (per serving):

- **Total calories:** 80

- **Protein:** 1g

- **Fiber content:** 2g

- **Carbs:** 20g

- **Fats:** 0g

Cinnamon-Spiced Applesauce

Time to Prepare: 10 minutes
Cook Time: 30 minutes
Number of Servings: 4

List of Ingredients:

- 4 medium apples, peeled, cored, and chopped (any variety)

- 1 cup of water

- 1 teaspoon of ground cinnamon

- 1/2 teaspoon of vanilla extract (optional)

- A pinch of nutmeg (optional)

Instructions:

1. In a medium saucepan, mix the chopped apples and water. Bring to a boil over medium heat.

2. Once boiling, reduce heat to low and cover. Simmer for about 20-30 minutes, or until the apples are soft.

3. Remove from heat and stir in the ground cinnamon, vanilla extract, and nutmeg (if using).

4. Use a potato masher or blender to puree the applesauce to your desired consistency (smooth or chunky).

5. Allow to cool slightly before serving. Store any leftovers in an airtight container in the refrigerator.

Nutritional Information (per serving):

- **Total calories:** 60

- **Protein:** 0g

- **Fiber content:** 2g

- **Carbs:** 15g

- **Fats:** 0g

Watermelon Slushie

Time to Prepare: 5 minutes
Cook Time: 0 minutes
Number of Servings: 2

List of Ingredients:

- 4 cups of seedless watermelon, cubed and frozen
- 1/4 cup of fresh mint leaves
- 1 tablespoon lime juice (optional)

Instructions:

1. In a blender, mix the frozen watermelon, fresh mint leaves, and lime juice (if using).
2. Blend on high speed until smooth and slushy, stopping to scrape down the sides as needed.
3. Taste and adjust sweetness or mintiness if desired by adding more mint or a splash of water.
4. Pour into glasses and serve immediately.

Nutritional Information (per serving):

- **Total calories:** 30
- **Protein:** 1g
- **Fiber content:** 1g
- **Carbs:** 7g
- **Fats:** 0g

Roasted Peaches with Vanilla Extract

Time to Prepare: 10 minutes
Cook Time: 15 minutes
Number of Servings: 4

List of Ingredients:

- 4 ripe peaches, halved and pitted
- 1 teaspoon of vanilla extract
- 1 teaspoon of cinnamon (optional)

Instructions:

1. Preheat the oven to 375°F (190°C).
2. Place the peach halves cut-side up in a baking dish.
3. Drizzle the vanilla extract over the peaches. Sprinkle with cinnamon if desired.
4. Roast in the oven for 15 minutes, until the peaches are tender and slightly caramelized.
5. Remove from the oven and let cool slightly before serving.

Nutritional Information (per serving):

- **Total calories:** 70
- **Protein:** 1g
- **Fiber content:** 2g
- **Carbs:** 17g
- **Fats:** 0g

Chilled Lemon and Berry Jelly

Time to Prepare: 10 minutes
Cook Time: 5 minutes
Number of Servings: 4

List of Ingredients:

- 1 cup of water
- 1 cup of fresh lemon juice
- 1 package (0.3 oz) sugar-free gelatin (lemon flavor)
- 1 cup of mixed berries (strawberries, blueberries, raspberries)

Instructions:

1. In a saucepan, bring 1 cup of water to a boil.
2. Remove from heat and stir in the sugar-free gelatin until fully dissolved.
3. Add the lemon juice and mix well.
4. Pour the mixture into a mold or individual serving cups of.
5. Add the mixed berries evenly into the gelatin mixture.
6. Refrigerate for at least 2 hours or until set.
7. Serve chilled.

Nutritional Information (per serving):

- **Total calories:** 30
- **Protein:** 1g
- **Fiber content:** 2g
- **Carbs:** 7g
- **Fats:** 0g

Orange and Grapefruit Segments with Fresh Mint

Time to Prepare: 10 minutes
Cook Time: 0 minutes
Number of Servings: 4

List of Ingredients:

- 2 large oranges, segmented
- 2 large grapefruits, segmented
- 1/4 cup of fresh mint leaves, chopped
- 1 tablespoon honey (optional, for sweetness)
- 1 tablespoon fresh lime juice

Instructions:

1. Peel the oranges and grapefruits, removing any white pith, and segment them over a bowl to catch any juices.
2. In a separate bowl, mix the honey (if using) and lime juice.
3. Add the mint leaves to the citrus segments and drizzle the lime-honey mixture over them.
4. Gently toss to mix all ingredients.
5. Serve immediately or chill in the refrigerator for 30 minutes before serving.

Nutritional Information (per serving):

- **Total calories:** 60
- **Protein:** 1g
- **Fiber content:** 3g
- **Carbs:** 14g
- **Fats:** 0g

CHAPTER 6: BEVERAGES

Cucumber Lemon Water

Time to Prepare: 5 minutes
Cook Time: 0 minutes
Number of Servings: 4

List of Ingredients:

- 1 medium cucumber, thinly sliced
- 1 lemon, thinly sliced
- 8 cups of water
- Fresh mint leaves (optional)

Instructions:

1. In a large pitcher, mix the cucumber and lemon slices.
2. Add the water and stir gently.
3. Let the mixture sit in the refrigerator for at least 1 hour to infuse the flavors.
4. Serve chilled, garnished with mint leaves if desired.

Nutritional Information (per serving):

- **Total calories:** 0
- **Protein:** 0g
- **Fiber content:** 0g
- **Carbs:** 0g
- **Fats:** 0g

Strawberry Mint Infused Water

Time to Prepare: 5 minutes
Cook Time: 0 minutes
Number of Servings: 4

List of Ingredients:

- 1 cup of fresh strawberries, hulled and sliced
- 1/4 cup of fresh mint leaves
- 8 cups of water

Instructions:

1. In a large pitcher, mix the sliced strawberries and mint leaves.

2. Pour in the water and stir gently to mix.
3. Let the mixture sit in the refrigerator for at least 1 hour to infuse the flavors.
4. Serve chilled.

Nutritional Information (per serving):

- **Total calories:** 0
- **Protein:** 0g
- **Fiber content:** 0g
- **Carbs:** 0g
- **Fats:** 0g

Green Detox Juice

Time to Prepare: 10 minutes
Cook Time: 0 minutes
Number of Servings: 2

List of Ingredients:

- 2 cups of kale leaves, stems removed
- 1 medium cucumber, chopped
- 1 green apple, cored and chopped
- Juice of 1 lemon
- 2 cups of water

Instructions:

1. In a blender, mix the kale, cucumber, green apple, lemon juice, and water.
2. Blend until smooth.
3. Strain the mixture through a fine mesh sieve or cheesecloth if desired for a smoother juice.
4. Serve immediately over ice or chill in the refrigerator.

Nutritional Information (per serving):

- **Total calories:** 50
- **Protein:** 2g
- **Fiber content:** 4g
- **Carbs:** 12g
- **Fats:** 0g

Spiced Ginger and Lemon Tea

Time to Prepare: 5 minutes
Cook Time: 10 minutes
Number of Servings: 2

List of Ingredients:

- 2 cups of water
- 1-inch piece fresh ginger, sliced
- Juice of 1 lemon
- 1-2 teaspoons of honey (optional)
- 1 cinnamon stick
- 2-3 whole cloves

Instructions:

1. In a saucepan, bring the water to a boil.
2. Add the sliced ginger, cinnamon stick, and cloves to the boiling water.
3. Reduce heat and let simmer for 10 minutes.
4. Remove from heat, strain into cups of, and stir in the lemon juice and honey if using.
5. Serve warm.

Nutritional Information (per serving):

- **Total calories:** 20
- **Protein:** 0g
- **Fiber content:** 0g
- **Carbs:** 5g
- **Fats:** 0g

Berry and Lime Sparkling Water

Time to Prepare: 5 minutes
Cook Time: 0 minutes
Number of Servings: 2

List of Ingredients:

- 1 cup of mixed berries (strawberries, blueberries, raspberries)
- Juice of 1 lime
- 2 cups of sparkling water
- Ice cubes (optional)
- Fresh mint leaves (for garnish, optional)

Instructions:

1. In a pitcher, muddle the mixed berries to release their juices.

2. Add the lime juice and mix well.
3. Pour in the sparkling water and stir gently.
4. Serve over ice, if desired, and garnish with mint leaves.

Nutritional Information (per serving):

- **Total calories:** 15
- **Protein:** 0g
- **Fiber content:** 1g
- **Carbs:** 4g
- **Fats:** 0g

Iced Hibiscus Tea with Fresh Lime

Time to Prepare: 10 minutes
Cook Time: 5 minutes
Number of Servings: 4

List of Ingredients:

- 4 cups of water
- 1/4 cup of dried hibiscus flowers
- Juice of 2 limes
- Lime slices (for garnish)
- Sweetener of choice (optional, to taste)
- Ice cubes

Instructions:

1. Boil the water in a pot.
2. Remove from heat and add the dried hibiscus flowers. Steep for about 5 minutes.
3. Strain the tea into a pitcher and let it cool.
4. Once cooled, stir in the lime juice. Sweeten if desired.
5. Serve over ice and garnish with lime slices.

Nutritional Information (per serving):

- **Total calories:** 10
- **Protein:** 0g
- **Fiber content:** 0g
- **Carbs:** 3g
- **Fats:** 0g

Watermelon Mint Cooler

Time to Prepare: 10 minutes
Cook Time: 0 minutes
Number of Servings: 4

List of Ingredients:

- 4 cups of seedless watermelon, cubed
- 1/4 cup of fresh mint leaves
- Juice of 1 lime
- 1 cup of ice cubes

Instructions:

1. In a blender, mix the watermelon cubes, fresh mint leaves, lime juice, and ice cubes.
2. Blend until smooth and frothy.
3. Pour into glasses and serve immediately, garnished with additional mint leaves if desired.

Nutritional Information (per serving):

- **Total calories:** 30
- **Protein:** 1g
- **Fiber content:** 1g
- **Carbs:** 8g
- **Fats:** 0g

Pineapple and Coconut Water Smoothie

Time to Prepare: 5 minutes
Cook Time: 0 minutes
Number of Servings: 2

List of Ingredients:

- 2 cups of fresh pineapple, chopped
- 1 cup of coconut water
- 1/2 cup of plain Greek yogurt (optional for creaminess)
- 1 cup of ice cubes

Instructions:

1. In a blender, mix the fresh pineapple, coconut water, and Greek yogurt (if using).
2. Add the ice cubes and blend until smooth and creamy.
3. Pour into glasses and serve immediately.

Nutritional Information (per serving):

- **Total calories:** 60
- **Protein:** 2g
- **Fiber content:** 1g
- **Carbs:** 14g
- **Fats:** 0g

Apple Cinnamon Iced Tea

Time to Prepare: 5 minutes
Cook Time: 10 minutes
Number of Servings: 4

List of Ingredients:

- 4 cups of water
- 4 apple-flavored herbal tea bags
- 1 cinnamon stick
- 1 medium apple, sliced
- Ice cubes

Instructions:

1. In a saucepan, bring the water to a boil. Remove from heat and add the tea bags and cinnamon stick.

2. Let steep for 5-7 minutes, then remove the tea bags and cinnamon stick.

3. Add the sliced apple to the tea and let it cool to room temperature.

4. Refrigerate for at least 1 hour or until chilled.

5. Serve over ice, with additional apple slices if desired.

Nutritional Information (per serving):

- **Total calories:** 10
- **Protein:** 0g
- **Fiber content:** 0g
- **Carbs:** 2g
- **Fats:** 0g

Citrus and Basil Sparkling Water

Time to Prepare: 5 minutes
Cook Time: 0 minutes
Number of Servings: 4

List of Ingredients:

- 1 lemon, sliced
- 1 orange, sliced
- 1 lime, sliced
- Fresh basil leaves (about 10 leaves)
- 4 cups of sparkling water
- Ice cubes

Instructions:

1. In a large pitcher, mix the lemon, orange, lime slices, and basil leaves.

2. Gently muddle the ingredients with a wooden spoon to release the citrus juices and basil aroma.

3. Fill glasses with ice cubes and pour the sparkling water over the mixture.

4. Stir gently and serve immediately. Garnish with additional basil leaves if desired.

Nutritional Information (per serving):

- **Total calories:** 0
- **Protein:** 0g
- **Fiber content:** 0g
- **Carbs:** 0g
- **Fats:** 0g

30-DAY MEAL PLAN

Day	Breakfast	Lunch	Snack	Dinner
1	Berry Bliss Yogurt Bowl	Mediterranean Chickpea Salad	Air-Fried Zucchini Chips	Lemon Garlic Chicken with Roasted Veggies
2	Veggie Omelet	Tuna and Cucumber Lettuce Wraps	Spiced Roasted Chickpeas	Baked Tilapia with Citrus Salsa
3	Apple Pie Oatmeal	Spicy Black Bean Soup	Baked Apple Chips	Zucchini Lasagna
4	Banana Pancakes	Zucchini Noodles with Tomato and Basil	Cucumber Slices with Salsa	Stuffed Bell Peppers with Ground Turkey
5	Cottage Cheese & Berry Parfait	Rainbow Veggie Wraps	Roasted Red Pepper Hummus with Veggie Sticks	Herb-Crusted Cod with Steamed Asparagus
6	Green Power Smoothie	Shrimp and Mango Salad	Hard-Boiled Eggs with Everything Seasoning	Turkey and Veggie Stir-Fry
7	Spinach and Tomato Egg Muffins	Cabbage Soup with Lean Turkey	Watermelon and Mint Salad	Cabbage and Carrot "Noodle" Pad Thai
8	Apple Cinnamon Breakfast Bake	Grilled Veggie Skewers with Lemon	Jicama Sticks with Lime and Chili	Eggplant and Tomato Bake
9	Mushroom and Asparagus Scramble	Spinach, Apple, and Walnut Salad	Cucumber Roll-Ups with Turkey Slices	Lemon Herb Shrimp with Broccoli
10	Mixed Berry Chia Pudding	Cucumber, Tomato, and Red Onion Salad	Tomato Basil Bites	Chili with Lean Ground Chicken
11	Tropical Fruit Salad	Butternut Squash Soup	Bell Pepper Nachos	Baked Spaghetti Squash with Marinara Sauce
12	Spiced Pumpkin Puree with Yogurt	Baked Bell Pepper and Tomato Casserole	Roasted Pumpkin Seeds	Cauliflower Fried Rice with Shrimp
13	Roasted Red Pepper and Spinach Egg White Cups	Roasted Cauliflower and Chickpea Bowl	Grilled Pineapple Rings with Cinnamon	Garlicky Spinach and Mushroom Sauté with Chicken
14	Banana-Berry Smoothie Bowl	Grilled Chicken Breast with Citrus Salad	Carrot and Celery Sticks with Greek Yogurt Dip	Spaghetti Squash and Turkey Meatballs
15	Pear and Ginger Smoothie	Chicken and Spinach Wrap	Air-Fried Zucchini Chips	Sweet and Spicy Baked Chicken Thighs

16	Baked Apple Slices with Cinnamon	Spicy Lentil and Tomato Soup	Spiced Roasted Chickpeas	Sautéed Shrimp with Zucchini and Squash Ribbons
17	Lemon and Blueberry Overnight Oats	Mushroom and Green Bean Stir-Fry	Cucumber Slices with Salsa	Mexican Cauliflower Rice with Black Beans
18	Grilled Peach and Greek Yogurt Bowl	Carrot and Ginger Soup	Bell Pepper Nachos	Dijin Mustard Chicken with Green Beans
19	Herb and Tomato Frittata	Roasted Tomato and Garlic Soup	Jicama Sticks with Lime and Chili	Eggplant and Tomato Bake
20	Berry Bliss Yogurt Bowl	Shrimp and Mango Salad	Mixed Berry Popsicles	Lemon Garlic Chicken with Roasted Veggies
21	Veggie Omelet	Mediterranean Chickpea Salad	Cucumber Roll-Ups with Turkey Slices	Grilled Salmon with Mango Salsa
22	Apple Pie Oatmeal	Tuna and Cucumber Lettuce Wraps	Hard-Boiled Eggs with Everything Seasoning	Baked Tilapia with Citrus Salsa
23	Banana Pancakes	Spicy Black Bean Soup	Roasted Red Pepper Hummus with Veggie Sticks	Zucchini Lasagna
24	Cottage Cheese & Berry Parfait	Zucchini Noodles with Tomato and Basil	Watermelon and Mint Salad	Stuffed Bell Peppers with Ground Turkey
25	Green Power Smoothie	Rainbow Veggie Wraps	Air-Fried Zucchini Chips	Turkey and Veggie Stir-Fry
26	Spinach and Tomato Egg Muffins	Cabbage Soup with Lean Turkey	Spiced Roasted Chickpeas	Garlic Herb Shrimp with Broccoli
27	Apple Cinnamon Breakfast Bake	Grilled Veggie Skewers with Lemon	Carrot and Celery Sticks	Sweet and Spicy Baked Chicken Thighs
28	Mushroom and Asparagus Scramble	Spinach, Apple, and Walnut Salad	Jicama Sticks with Lime and Chili	Baked Spaghetti Squash with Marinara Sauce
29	Mixed Berry Chia Pudding	Cucumber, Tomato, and Red Onion Salad	Tomato Basil Bites	Chili with Lean Ground Chicken
30	Tropical Fruit Salad	Roasted Cauliflower and Chickpea Bowl	Bell Pepper Nachos	Grilled Chicken Breast with Citrus Salad

MEASUREMENT CONVERSION TABLE

Measurement	Imperial (US)	Metric
Volume		
1 teaspoon	1 teaspoon	5 milliliters
1 tablespoon	1 tablespoon	15 milliliters
1 fluid ounce	1 fl oz	30 milliliters
1 cup	1 cup	240 milliliters
1 pint	1 pt	473 milliliters
1 quart	1 qt	0.95 liters
1 gallon	1 gal	3.8 liters
Weight		
1 ounce	1 oz	28 grams
1 pound	1 lb	454 grams
Temperature		
32°F	32°F	0°C
212°F	212°F	100°C
Other		
1 stick of butter	1 stick	113 grams

CONCLUSION

Congratulations on finishing this Weight Watchers Zero Point Weight Loss Cookbook! We hope these tasty and nutritious recipes have encouraged you to adopt a lifestyle of balanced eating and thoughtful choices. Remember that improving your health involves more than just what you eat; it's also about the habits you create and the happiness you discover in caring for your body.

You can enjoy tasty meals and snacks that satisfy your cravings and help you stick to your weight loss goals. Every recipe in this collection is made to be straightforward, easy to follow, and flexible, giving you the chance to express your creativity in the kitchen.

As you move forward on your health journey, pay attention to your body, acknowledge your achievements, and have fun along the way. Share these recipes with your friends and family to inspire them to make healthier choices too.

I am grateful that you have chosen this cookbook to be a part of your journey. Here's to your health, happiness, and a plethora of delicious meals ahead! Enjoy your cooking!

RECIPES INDEX

Orange and Grapefruit Segments with Fresh Mint 60

Pear and Ginger Smoothie 16

Pineapple and Coconut Water Smoothie 63

Rainbow Veggie Wraps 21

Roasted Cauliflower and Chickpea Bowl 25

Roasted Peaches with Vanilla Extract 59

Roasted Pumpkin Seeds 52

Roasted Red Pepper and Spinach Egg White Cups 15

Roasted Red Pepper Hummus with Veggie Sticks 48

Roasted Tomato and Eggplant Stew 42

Roasted Tomato and Garlic Soup 27

Shrimp and Mango Salad 21

Spiced Ginger and Lemon Tea 62

Spiced Pumpkin Puree with Yogurt 14

Spiced Roasted Chickpeas 47

Spicy Black Bean Soup 20

Spicy Lentil and Tomato Soup 28

Spicy Pickled Veggies 54

Spinach and Tomato Egg Muffins 12

Spinach, Apple, and Walnut Salad 23

Strawberry Mango Sorbet 58

Strawberry Mint Infused Water 61

Stuffed Bell Peppers with Ground Turkey 32

Sweet and Sour Cabbage Slaw 26

Sweet and Spicy Baked Chicken Thighs 46

Tomato Basil Bites 51

Tropical Fruit Salad 14

Tuna and Cucumber Lettuce Wraps 19

Turkey and Veggie Stir-Fry 34

Veggie Omelet 9

Watermelon and Mint Salad 49

Watermelon Mint Cooler 63

Watermelon Slushie 59

Zucchini Lasagna (using zucchini slices as "noodles") 31

Zucchini Noodles with Tomato and Basil 20

Printed in Great Britain
by Amazon